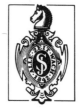

Treatment in Clinical Medicine

Series Editor: John L. Reid

Titles in the series already published:

Gastrointestinal Disease
Edited by C.J.C. Roberts

Rheumatic Disease
Hilary A. Capell, T.J. Daymond
and W. Carson Dick

Forthcoming titles in the series:

Cardiovascular Disease
A.R. Lorimer and W. Stewart Hillis

Neurological and Neuro-psychiatric Disorders
J.D. Parkes, P. Jenner, D. Rushton and C.D. Marsden

Hypertension
B.N.C. Prichard and C.W.I. Owens

Respiratory Disease
Anne E. Tattersfield and M. McNicol

W.J. MacLennan · A.N. Shepherd
I.H. Stevenson

The Elderly

With 33 Figures

Springer-Verlag
Berlin Heidelberg New York Tokyo 1984

W.J. MacLennan, MD, FRCP (Glas., Ed., Lond.)
Senior Lecturer in Geriatric Medicine, University Department of
Medicine, Ninewells Hospital and Medical School, Dundee DD1
9SY, Scotland

A.N. Shepherd, BSc, MRCP (UK)
Lecturer in Medicine, University Department of Medicine,
Ninewells Hospital and Medical School, Dundee DD1 9SY,
Scotland

I.H. Stevenson, BSc, PhD
Professor of Pharmacology, Department of Pharmacology and
Clinical Pharmacology, Ninewells Hospital and Medical School,
Dundee DD1 9SY, Scotland

Series Editor:
John L. Reid, MD, FRCP
Regius Professor of Materia Medica,
University of Glasgow, Scotland

ISBN 3-540-13236-8 Springer-Verlag Berlin Heidelberg New York Tokyo
ISBN 0-387-13236-8 Springer-Verlag New York Heidelberg Berlin Tokyo

Typeset by Latimer Trend & Company Ltd, Plymouth
Printed by Page Bros. (Norwich) Ltd, Mile Cross Lane, Norwich

2128/3916-543210

Series Editor's Foreword

"The Elderly" is the third monograph in a series on management and treatment in major patient groups and subspecialties. Each book is complete in its own right. The whole series, however, has been prepared to fill a gap between standard text-books of medicine and therapeutics and research reviews, symposia and original articles in specialist fields. The aim of the series is to present up-to-date authoritative advice on patient management with particular reference to drug treatment. The first two volumes in the series, on gastrointestinal diseases and rheumatic diseases, were addressed to major therapeutic areas or subspecialties. The present volume, "The Elderly", is intended to provide overall guidance on the management of a range of medical problems in elderly patients. The elderly make up an increasing proportion of the population and require a substantial proportion of health care resources. The management of elderly patients falls not only upon specialist geriatricians but also upon a range of others, including general practitioners, general physicians and almost all other medical specialists with the exception of paediatricians.

It has become apparent in recent years that the management of disease in the elderly in general and drug treatment in particular presents new problems and challenges. Some of these relate to the wide spectrum of disease in elderly patients, in whom there is often multiple pathology, while others concern age-induced changes in drug handling or drug effect. It is appropriate that the authors of the volume on The Elderly are from Dundee, where much of the basic and applied clinical research in this area has been undertaken in recent years. Drs MacLennan and Shepherd and Professor Stevenson bring their own individual experience as geriatrician, physician and pharmacologist respectively, to provide a multidisciplinary input to the volume. In the first chapter there is a detailed review of the effects of ageing on drug handling and action. It is followed by a review of practical problems and then a system by system account of common diseases and problems presenting in the elderly. In particular, there are chapters on the management of bladder disorders and on terminal care and long-term care. These subjects, while presenting frequent management difficulties, are rarely reviewed in standard texts.

The aim of the series is to present clinical and therapeutic approaches in the context of developments in clinical pharmacology. I believe this has been successfully achieved in this volume, as the theoretical mechanisms are balanced by discussion of the practical problems. The volumes are intended to be guides to treatment and to assist in the choice of drug regimen. They should provide easy reference to drug interactions and adverse reactions. It should be particularly useful for the young hospital doctor in training for higher qualifications. However, it is likely that the present volume will be of value to senior medical students and to those in established posts in hospital or general practice who are seeking to update their knowledge and to view developments in the care of the elderly.

Glasgow, May 1984   John L. Reid

Preface

In developed countries the elderly population has increased markedly over the last half century and is likely to continue to do so for the next two decades. Multiple pathology is common in this age group with degenerative and chronic disease being particularly prevalent. As a result, drug prescribing is disproportionately high in the elderly and often involves the administration of several drugs concurrently. Adverse reactions, whether stemming from increased drug use, increased pharmacological response or impairment of homoeostatic mechanisms, have been shown to occur more frequently in elderly patients. Appropriate drug treatment in the elderly is therefore obviously of considerable importance both in patient management and in economic terms.

Few texts deal specifically with drug therapy in the elderly and this volume is intended to cover disorders where the treatment varies either qualitatively or quantitatively from that in younger patients. Some diseases are peculiar to the elderly and have particular significance in that age group. In some cases specific drugs or drug groups are unsuitable for the elderly patient or may require greater supervision; in other cases simple adjustment of dosage may suffice. Disease and the effect of ageing often enhance the effects of drugs in old age. Taking into account the potential adverse effects of many drugs when given to the elderly it is hoped that this text will encourage the prescriber to set and observe identifiable therapeutic goals.

There are many pharmacological reasons for differences in drug response in the elderly and a chapter is devoted to general consideration of altered pharmacokinetic facts, i.e. of drug absorption, distribution, metabolism, and excretion. The present state of knowledge of possible alteration in pharmacodynamics is discussed, although it is difficult to unravel the complexities of altered homoeostasis and end organ sensitivity in relation to the ageing process in the presence of both overt and possibly covert disease. Pharmacokinetic information on individual drugs, where clinically important, is to be found in the general text.

Chapters are linked to the systems of the body with, in each case, definition of the drugs and drug groups that are particularly applicable. Some sections are deliberately short where drug treatment does not vary significantly from that in younger patients.

The volume is intended to meet not only the needs of specialists in geriatric medicine but also those of general physicians and general practitioners who inevitably are faced with therapeutic problems in the older age group.

Acknowledgement

We are extremely grateful to Maureen Hughes for all the time and effort she put into organising the figures, tables and index, and for typing the manuscript.

Contents

1 The Effect of Ageing on Pharmacokinetics and Pharmacodynamics

In the last decade there has been a marked increase of interest in the clinical pharmacology of old age and publications on this topic have increased quite spectacularly during the period. This new interest in the elderly has arisen for three main reasons—the considerable growth in the elderly population, their disproportionately high drug use, and most particularly, the increased incidence of adverse drug effects in this age group.

Drug Use and Adverse Drug Reactions in Elderly Populations

In developed countries, the proportion of old people is increasing. Population data from the United Kingdom and the United States show the number of people of 65 years and over to be increasing, both in absolute terms and as a proportion of the total population. According to demographic predictions, the elderly population in the UK will reach a peak of 8.2 millions in the early 1990s from a starting point of 5.4 millions in 1961.

In addition to constituting an increasing population, the elderly receive more drugs than younger age groups and consequently drug use by this age group is of considerable economic as well as medical importance. In the UK the elderly, comprising some 12% of the population in 1975, were responsible for 21% of the National Health Service expenditure on prescriptions. In the United States in 1976, the 10% of the population who were elderly spent more than 20% of the national total drug budget.

A number of studies have demonstrated that the elderly are more at risk of developing adverse drug reactions, a finding perhaps not unexpected in view of the multiple pathology occurring in the age group and the frequent need therefore to use several drugs concurrently.

With a number of individual drugs, the incidence of adverse reactions has also been reported to increase with age. The Boston Collaborative Drug Surveillance Program has demonstrated a clear relationship between age and adverse effects of heparin and of several benzodiazepines—chlordiazepoxide, diazepam, flurazepam, and nitrazepam. The benzodiazepines produced mainly unwanted central nervous system depression and the effects were clearly dose-related, the age-related trend being absent at lower doses. Furthermore, the vast majority of reactions occurred within the first 3 days of starting therapy. For the cardiac drugs lignocaine and propranolol they reported a relatively weak association between age and clinical toxicity and commented that for some 90 other drugs in common clinical use, age alone was not a major determinant of clinical toxicity.

Different patterns of adverse drug reactions occur outside hospital, there being additional factors to be considered, such as the misuse of drugs by the elderly through non-compliance. When the large number of drugs prescribed for the elderly is considered in combination with their increased susceptibility to adverse drug reactions, it becomes apparent that probably more than half of all unwanted drug effects occur in geriatric patients.

Determinants of Altered Drug Response in the Elderly

There is now a considerable body of evidence to indicate that the response to many drugs may change as people age. The three principal factors contributing to such age-related alterations in pharmacodynamics are:

1) Altered pharmacokinetics
2) Change in receptor sensitivity or density
3) Impairment of normal homoeostatic mechanisms

A fourth factor of difficulty in older age groups of complying with prescribing instructions is of considerable importance and is dealt with in Chap. 2. The alteration in response to a drug may be multifactorial, involving a complex interplay between the three factors listed. Disease is very often present and it is difficult to separate age effects per se from those resulting from ageing associated with the presence of pathological change. The elderly, while referred to collectively, are a heterogeneous group ranging from "fit old folk" to the grossly debilitated. Patients admitted to geriatric units usually have evidence of multiple pathology and the consequent need to prescribe several drugs concurrently makes the conduct and interpretation of drug studies in the elderly difficult. Changes, as people age, in social habits such as patterns of activity, smoking habits, and alcohol consumption are further complicating factors.

Pharmacokinetics

Drug kinetics in the elderly may conveniently be considered under the headings of absorption, distribution, hepatic metabolism (including pre-systemic elimination), and renal excretion.

Drug Absorption

Table 1.1 summarises changes occurring in gastro-intestinal physiology with age together with the main pharmacokinetic findings to date. There are a number of changes in the gastro-intestinal tract in the elderly which might be expected to alter oral drug absorption, e.g. increased pH consequent upon decreased gastric acid output, decreased intestinal blood flow secondary to decreased cardiac output, and alterations in gastric emptying time and gastro-intestinal motility. It is perhaps surprising therefore that for a great many drugs, the available evidence indicates that the rate and extent of drug absorption are largely unchanged in the elderly. Attention should be drawn however to the inadequacy of much of the pharmacokinetic data, obtained in many cases from the early phase of drug elimination studies and with limited blood sampling over the absorption period. In addition, few studies have compared intravenous and plasma drug concentration versus time profiles in the two age groups.

Table 1.1. Drug absorption in old age—changes in gastro-intestinal physiology and pharmacokinetic consequences[a]

Physiological changes	Drugs which appear to be absorbed normally in the elderly	Drugs which appear to be absorbed less rapidly or to a lesser extent
↓ gastric pH (due to acid output) ↓ gastro-intestinal motility ↓ gastro-intestinal blood flow ↓ mucosal cell absorbing area	Aspirin, ampicillin, antipyrine, dextropropoxyphene, indomethacin, lithium, lorazepam, morphine, paracetamol, pivmecillinam, quinine, sulphamethizole, tetracycline, theophylline	Chlordiazepoxide, digoxin, levodopa, metoprolol, propicillin, prazosin

[a] Sources of pharmacokinetic information: Stevenson et al. (1980) and Koch-Weser et al. (1982)

Changes where they do occur are often small and unlikely to be of clinical significance, particularly during chronic therapy. With digoxin and theophylline for example, the extent of absorption determined by comparison of oral and intravenous plasma drug concentration profiles was similar in the two age groups and the sole difference was a delay in the absorption of digoxin in the elderly group of patients studied. As will be discussed in the section on hepatic drug metabolism and pre-systemic elimination, age-related changes in absorption are likely to be of greatest significance where there is a reduced first-pass effect in the elderly. With a drug such as levodopa, both a reduced first-pass effect and a more rapid gastric emptying with reduced gastric degradation are responsible for the greater area under the curve (AUC) in the elderly. After oral dosing, plasma drug concentration and AUC are often higher in elderly subjects than in young controls. However in almost all cases these changes are likely to result from impairment of metabolism (e.g. aspirin, chlormethiazole, metoprolol, propranolol, and paracetamol), decreased renal excretion (propicillin, procaine), or a reduction in distribution volume (quinine, antipyrine) rather than from increased absorption. The only drug for which there is good evidence (from oral/intravenous comparison) of a substantial reduction in extent of absorption is prazosin, the bio-availability of which in the elderly has been shown to be only some 60% of that in younger subjects in the absence of any alteration in extent of first-pass metabolism, suggesting that the grastrointestinal absorption of prazosin decreases in old age.

Drug Distribution

Table 1.2 summarises the physiological changes occurring with ageing which are likely to influence a drug's distribution in the body, together with the principal pharmacokinetic findings.

Table 1.2. Drug distribution in old age—physiological changes and pharmacokinetic consequences[a]

Physiological changes	Pharmacokinetic consequences
↓ lean body mass ↓ total body water ↑ body fat ↓ plasma albumin ↓ membrane integrity?	No change in distribution volume of some drugs—phenylbutazone, sulphamethizole, warfarin ↓ volume of distribution of some hydrophilic drugs—antipyrine, quinine, paracetamol, ethanol ↑ volume of distribution of some lipophilic drugs—diazepam, lignocaine ↓ extent of plasma protein binding of some drugs—pethidine, phenytoin, carbenoxolone, tolbutamide, temazepam ↑ binding to red cells—pethidine ↑ penetration of drugs e.g. through blood-brain barrier—nitrazepam (rat study)

[a] Sources of pharmacokinetic information: Crooks et al. (1976) and Vestal (1978)

The most important features of a drug's distribution are distribution in body fluids and the extent of binding to plasma proteins (usually to albumin but with some drugs to alpha₁ acid glycoprotein), to red cells and to body tissues, including the target organ. In old age there is a significant decrease in lean body mass and total body water, an increase in body fat (particularly in males) and a small but significant decrease in plasma albumin. While it is difficult to generalise, the distribution of hydrophilic drugs such as antipyrine, quinine, and paracetamol may decrease in the elderly whereas lipophilic drugs such as lignocaine, chlordiazepoxide, and, in particular, diazepam appear to be more extensively distributed. Differences in body composition between men and women, irrespective of age, may be as profound as those between the young and the elderly, with the distribution of lipophilic drugs being more extensive in women.

Overall, the elderly are smaller in body size than younger subjects and this may contribute in part, for example, to the higher blood levels of many drugs in the elderly following the same dose to young and elderly patients. This could therefore provide a relatively simple explanation of the exaggerated effects of some drugs in elderly patients.

Plasma albumin concentrations are slightly lower in healthy old people than in their younger counterparts and may be markedly so in the poorly nourished or severely debilitated elderly. This will result in an increase in the free pharmacologically active fraction of some drugs and in turn lead to a greater distribution and, with some drugs, a more rapid elimination. There is also some evidence to suggest that in the elderly, drugs may be more readily displaced from plasma protein binding sites by other drugs, partly as a consequence of the reduced plasma protein concentrations.

The extent of plasma protein binding of phenytoin, carbenoxolone, and temazepam is slightly reduced in the elderly. On the other hand, no detectable alteration occurs in the plasma protein binding of diazepam and with warfarin the evidence is contradictory. The practical significance of such changes in distribution volume and extent of protein binding is unclear, but they are of major importance in the interpretation of other pharmacokinetic data, such as drug plasma half-life. It is doubtful whether changes in protein binding are of great clinical importance, although the possibility of such changes influencing, or reflecting alteration in, a drug's penetration to its site of action cannot be excluded. One study has demonstrated a greater penetration of ^{14}C-nitrazepam into the brain of elderly rats in the absence of any other age-related pharmacokinetic differences and may reflect a loss of the integrity of the blood-brain barrier with ageing.

Drug Elimination

Drug elimination involves the two linked processes of hepatic metabolism (whereby most drugs are converted to more polar metabolites) and renal excretion (the excretion by the kidney of polar drugs and metabolites). The physiological changes occurring in these processes with ageing are summarised in Table 1.3 together with the main pharmacokinetic consequences. The only valid parameter in assessing age-related differences in drug disposition is that of clearance, since elimination half-life may be markedly affected by distribution changes associated with ageing.

In the earliest study of drug metabolism in relation to age, the hepatic clearance of antipyrine, a drug widely used as an index of liver microsomal oxidation, was shown to be reduced in the elderly. This would seem to be partly due to an age-related decrease in functional liver volume and partly to a reduced rate of hepatic metabolism. Several other drugs undergoing oxidation exhibit a similar reduction in clearance (e.g. chlordiazepoxide, theophylline, nortripty-

Table 1.3 Drug elimination in old age—changes in hepatic and renal physiology and pharmacokinetic consequences[a]

Physiological changes	Pharmacokinetic consequences
(i) Hepatic function ↓ hepatic size ↓ hepatic blood flow ↓ number of functional cells ↓ microsomal enzyme activity	(i) *Metabolised drugs* No appreciable change in clearance of ethanol, oxazepam, flunitrazepam, lorazepam, nitrazepam, temazepam, isoniazid, metoprolol, digitoxin, prazosin ↓ clearance of antipyrine, chlordiazepoxide, desmethyldiazepam, theophylline, nortriptyline ↓ first-pass extraction and ↑ bio-availability of chlormethiazole, labetalol, propranolol, lignocaine
(ii) Renal function ↓ renal blood flow ↓ glomerular filtration ↓ tubular excretion	(ii) *Drugs excreted unchanged* ↓ elimination of penicillin, dihydrostreptomycin, tetracycline, kanamycin, digoxin, practolol, sulphamethizole, phenobarbitone

[a] Sources of pharmacokinetic information: Crooks et al. (1976) and Koch-Weser et al. (1982)

line) but for some other oxidised drugs (e.g. warfarin, digitoxin, prazosin) no age-related differences in clearance exist. It is apparent therefore that there is no simple pattern of age-related change in drug metabolism. Changes, where they occur, are often small and may be less important than those brought about by environmental factors such as smoking. The individual's sex is an additional factor and the sex differences which occur in the disposition of some drugs seem to reduce with ageing. Even within a single group of drugs such as the benzodiazepines, age-related changes in metabolism are inconsistent and are influenced by metabolic route and by distribution volume of the individual drug. In general, age-related differences in metabolism occur to a greater extent with benzodiazepines undergoing oxidative metabolism rather than conjugation.

A complicating factor in many studies on drug metabolism is the presence of disease or hospitalisation of the population under study. In a recent investigation on benoxaprofen, Hosie and Stevenson (personal communication) reported a mean half-life of 47 h in a group of elderly arthritic out-patients, i.e. a figure much closer to the value of 26 h in healthy younger subjects than the values of 111 and 101 h for elderly hospitalised patients from other studies.

A number of drugs are so avidly extracted by the liver, i.e. by uptake into hepatic binding sites and by metabolism, and that their clearance depends on rate of delivery to the liver in the blood. In old age, a decrease in hepatic blood flow together with possible reduction in the rate of hepatic metabolism is responsible for the reduced elimination of such high-clearance drugs as chlormethiazole, labetalol, lignocaine, and possibly propranolol, although the evidence on the last-named is conflicting. With such high-clearance drugs there is a marked first-pass effect due to their extensive pre-systemic removal from the blood on their first passage through the liver. Their oral bio-availability is therefore low but is increased in the elderly due to a reduction in the first-pass extraction.

Drug-metabolising ability may be enhanced by treatment with enzyme-inducing agents such as phenobarbitone or phenytoin or by exposure to environmental factors such as cigarette smoking. While no conclusive data exist, there is some evidence to suggest that the induction response may be reduced in the elderly. If this were the case, the elderly as well as having a lower baseline ability to metabolise some drugs would be less able to develop tolerance to metabolised drugs.

The effects of age on renal function exert a profound influence on the elimination of a number of drugs. In many cases, drugs are excreted by simple glomerular filtration and their rate of excretion correlates with glomerular filtration rate (and hence with creatinine clearance), e.g. digoxin and the aminoglycoside antibiotics. In old age, renal function diminishes consequent on reduced renal blood flow, so that at age 65 there is a reduction of approximately 30% in glomerular filtration rate compared with young adults. Tubular function also deteriorates with age and drugs such as penicillin and procainamide which are actively secreted by renal tubules show a marked reduction in clearance.

Where there is obvious renal disease, guidance for appropriate dosage of renally excreted drugs may be obtained from standard tables. With some drugs this is particularly important because of the serious effects of overdosage, e.g. digoxin, lithium, aminoglycoside antibiotics, and chlorpropamide. In general, elderly patients are best treated with lower doses of renally excreted drugs than are younger patients.

Much of the pharmacokinetic data on hepatic metabolism and renal excretion of drugs in the elderly has been obtained from single-dose studies and there is a paucity of data on age-related comparisons of steady-state drug levels with chronic dosing. With renally excreted drugs such as digoxin, penicillin, and streptomycin, adequate serum levels are obtained in the elderly with lower doses. Elderly patients have also been shown to require lower doses of lithium salts to maintain similar plasma levels and efficacy to those in their younger counterparts. With metabolised drugs it is again not possible to generalise. Plasma steady-state levels of propranolol and phenytoin increase with age, as do those of some, but not all, tricyclic antidepressants. In a recent chronic-dose study, Hosie and Stevenson (personal communication) measured steady-state plasma levels of benoxaprofen in a group of elderly arthritic patients and showed that, once steady state was reached after a few days' treatment, no further accumulation occurred during the 20 weeks of the study.

In general, drug elimination is often reduced in the elderly, particularly in the sick elderly. This occurs most consistently with drugs eliminated by renal mechanism where the extent of the reduction is such that, without adjustment of dose, excessive drug accumulation and toxicity may result. With drugs which are metabolised, the situation is less definite, but the rate of metabolism of some drugs is appreciably slower in older age groups. The situation is complicated, however, by dietary and smoking habits and by the presence of disease. With drugs undergoing first-pass elimination, there may be a marked increase in bio-availability of the first dose and exaggerated effects may be seen.

Change in Receptor Sensitivity or Density

Despite the presence of many differences in drug handling which help to account for variations in drug effects between the old and the young, there is still, as summarised in Table 1.4, a significant residue of altered responsiveness which seems to be explicable only by differences in tissue "sensitivity" to drugs. It is obviously not possible in most cases to measure true receptor sensitivity and most studies simply related drug effect to the dose required or to the plasma drug concentration at which the effect occurred. Elderly patients would seem to be more sensitive to the anticoagulant effect of warfarin than their younger counterparts since, at the same plasma concentration, there is greater inhibition of vitamin-K-dependent clotting factor synthesis in elderly than in younger patients. The innovative studies reported by Castleden et al. (1977) indicated an increased sensitivity of the elderly central nervous system to nitrazepam in that single doses impaired psychomotor performance in the elderly to a greater extent than in the young, in the absence of any age-related pharmacokinetic differences. Similar findings have subsequently been reported for the hypnotics temazepam and chlormethiazole but to a lesser extent for diazepam and dichloralphenazone. The elderly have also been reported to be more sensitive to the depressant effects of diazepam, as indicated by the plasma concentration to achieve sedation in patients being premedicated for elective cardioversion and by dose requirements for intubation in patients undergoing endoscopy.

Several studies have implicated alteration in beta-adrenoceptor sensitivity in old age, there being an age-related increase in the dose of isoprenaline required to induce tachycardia and a decrease in the extent of blockade of the isoprenaline-induced tachycardia by propranolol. These effects may be related to a reduction in the number of receptors with increasing age, some evidence for which has been provided from studies of beta-adrenoceptor density on human lymphocytes.

Table 1.4. Alterations in drug response in old age occurring in the absence of pharmacokinetic change[a]

Drug	Effect in old age
Warfarin	↑ anticoagulant effect
Nitrazepam	↑ impairment of performance
Diazepam	↓ dose for CNS depression
Diazepam	↓ dose for intubation
Diazepam	↑ body sway
Temazepam	↑ body sway and reaction time. ↓ CNS arousal
Chlormethiazole	↑ body sway and reaction time. ↓ CNS arousal
Dichloralphenazone	↑ body sway
Isoprenaline	↑ dose for tachycardia
Propranolol	↑ dose for block of isoprenaline induced tachycardia
Propranolol	↑ dose for block of exercise induced tachycardia

[a] Sources of information: Vestal (1978), Crooks and Stevenson (1981), and Stevenson (1983)

Impairment of Normal Homoeostatic Mechanism

Drug "sensitivity" may also be altered by the presence of disease, either directly by the pathological processes commonly found in the elderly or indirectly by associated complications such as peripheral circulatory failure, anaemia, poor nutrition, or hepatic, cardiac, and renal failure. The increased risk of haemorrhagic complications of anticoagulants in the elderly is, in part at least, due to degenerative vascular disease diminishing the homoeostatic response. Other homoeostatic mechanisms are also considerably blunted in geriatric patients. Drug-induced postural hypotension is particularly evident in this age group and many non-specific unwanted drug effects in the elderly, such as dizziness, confusion, agitation, weakness, altered bowel habit, etc., may reflect effects that in the younger patient would be prevented by more efficient homoeostatic mechanisms. Drugs used in the treatment of hypertension and diuretics, especially thiazides, carry a particularly high risk of postural hypotension.

The elderly have an impaired thermoregulatory capacity and several psychoactive drugs commonly prescribed for the elderly may precipitate hypothermia, partly through a direct pharmacological effect, but also indirectly through reduction in physical activity.

Other homoeostatic mechanisms which may be less efficient in old age and therefore result in increased "sensitivity" to the adverse effects of a variety of drugs include the regulation of blood sugar levels and the neurological control of bladder and bowel function.

As previously referred to, elderly patients often show an exaggerated response to single doses of a number of benzodiazepine hypnotics and adverse effects might be anticipated with chronic use in view of the tendency of such drugs to accumulate in the elderly. Interestingly, a recent community study has shown no appreciable impairment of mental function in elderly patients on long-term therapy with nitrazepam or flurazepam. The findings indicate therefore that adaptation of the central nervous system to chronic benzodiazepine therapy may occur in the elderly.

The response to many drugs undoubtedly changes as people age as a result of a complex alteration, with ageing, of pharmacokinetic processes, sensitivity factors, and physiological homoeostatic mechanisms. Of the pharmacokinetic changes, decreased renal elimination and a reduced first-pass extraction resulting in increased drug bio-availability are particularly important. In the case of tissue sensitivity, there have been few opportunities so far to determine age-related changes in the number and sensitivity of drug receptors and studies have been largely confined to relating drug effects to plasma levels in patients of different age.

Such investigations have been complicated by the presence of disease in the elderly populations under study and it is difficult to differentiate between age effects per se and those associated with disease. In the evaluation of new drugs it will be essential to obtain a comprehensive database from which drug regimens appropriate for elderly patients may be developed.

References

Castleden CM, George CF, Marcer D, Hallet C (1977) Increased sensitivity to nitrazepam in old age. Br Med J 1: 10–12

Crooks J, O'Malley K, Stevenson IH (1976) Pharmacokinetics in the elderly. Clin Pharmacokin 1: 280–296

Crooks J, Stevenson IH (1979) Drugs and the elderly, Macmillan, London

Crooks J, Stevenson IH (1981) Drug response in the elderly—sensitivity and pharmacokinetic considerations. Age Ageing 10: 73–80

Koch-Weser J, Greenblatt DJ, Sellers EM, Shader RI (1982) Drug disposition in old age. New Engl J Med 306: 1081–1086

O'Malley K, Judge TG, Crooks J (1980) Geriatric clinical pharmacology and therapeutics. In: Avery GS (ed) Drug treatment, Adis Press, Australia

Stevenson IH, Salem SAM, O'Malley K, Cusack B, Kelly JG (1980) In: Prescott LF, Nimmo WS (eds) Drug absorption, Adis Press, New York, pp 253–261

Stevenson IH (1984) Proceedings 2nd World Conference on Clinical Pharmacology and Therapeutics (in press)

Swift CG, Stevenson IH (1983) Benzodiazepines in the elderly. In: Costa E (ed) The benzodiazepines, Raven Press, pp 225–236

Vestal RE (1978) Drug use in the elderly: a review of problems and special considerations. Drugs 16: 358–382

Vestal RE, Wood AJJ, Shand DG (1979) Reduced β-adrenoreceptor sensitivity in the elderly. Clin Pharmacol Ther 26: 181–186

2 Practical Problems

Multiple Pathology, Polypharmacy, and Drug Compliance

On first meeting an elderly patient, a doctor often is faced with the dilemma of deciding which of the many disorders he identified should be treated. When Wilson et al. (1962) reviewed 200 patients admitted to a geriatric unit they found that each, on average, suffered from six different diseases. The number of these rose with patient age (Fig. 2.1). Disorders most frequently contributing to multiple pathology were cerebrovascular disease, pneumonia, urinary infection, ischaemic or hypertensive heart disease, dementia, chronic bronchitis, cataract, pressure sores, normochromic anaemia, renal failure, cancer, and prostatic enlargement (Fig. 2.2).

From such a pattern it requires little imagination to picture an elderly woman admitted to hospital with stroke in whom further enquiry reveals there has been a long history of hypertension complicated by congestive cardiac failure and chronic uraemia. In addition to contributing to her cardiac and cerebrovascular disease, heavy smoking has left her with chronic bronchitis. Since she had fallen and lain on the floor overnight she has a bronchopneumonia, and is beginning to develop a sacral pressure sore. Neighbours give a story that she has been behaving oddly for some time and it is obvious from cursory examination that she is very agitated. Routine laboratory investigation reveals that she has a normochromic normocytic anaemia, probably associated with her chronic uraemia.

In such a situation the doctor might prescribe naftidrofuryl to improve her cerebral blood flow; a large dose of methyldopa to reduce her blood pressure; digoxin, frusemide, and potassium supplements to control her cardiac failure; salbutamol to prevent bronchospasm; ascorbic acid and zinc sulphate to promote healing of her pressure area; amoxycillin to treat her pneumonia; and large regular doses of chlorpromazine to control her agitation. Attacked by such a regime it is likely that if the patient does not die from one of her many diseases she will succumb to either the side-effects of one of the drugs, or from interactions between several of them.

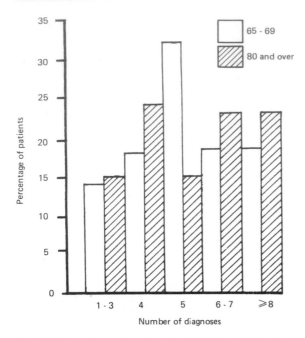

Fig. 2.1. Percentages of patients aged 65–69 and 80 and over related to number of diagnoses in individual patients (Wilson et al. 1962).

A doctor adopting this approach requires guidelines fundamental to successful drug therapy in the elderly (Table 2.1). If he had used these he would have recognised that chlorpromazine might interact with methyldopa to produce profound hypotension; and if using methyldopa at all would have started with the smallest dose possible. He also would have recognised the dangers of polypharmacy and thus started by only using drugs which were essential. Thus medication might have been limited in the present case to frusemide and amoxycillin. A more critical evaluation of the agitation would have revealed that this was due to a faecal impaction and that an enema rather than a tranquilliser was the appropriate approach. Hypotensive drugs are unlikely to

Table 2.1. Guidelines for prescribing in the elderly (Hall 1973)

1. Know pharmacology of drug used
2. Use lowest dose likely to be effective
3. Use fewest drugs required
4. Identify cause of symptoms before treatment
5. Do not continue a drug if it is no longer necessary
6. Do not use a cure that is worse than the disease
7. Do not withhold drugs on account of old age

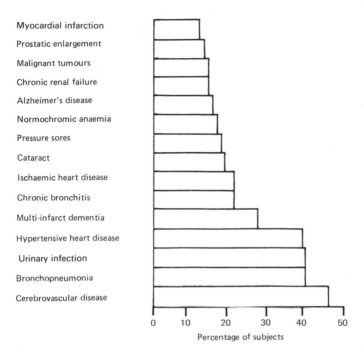

Fig. 2.2. Percentages of subjects suffering from particular diagnoses (Wilson et al. 1962).

prevent recurrence of a stroke, so that the drowsiness and depression associated with methyldopa would have been worse than any marginal reduction of risk it conferred. Again, once the condition of the patient was stabilised it would have been worth considering whether the diuretic which she had taken for 5 years should be discontinued. Our hypothetical doctor is unlikely to have been deterred from prescribing, but if the patient had been in atrial fibrillation, had not been hypotensive, and had given a history to suggest cerebral embolism, anticoagulants should not have been withheld merely on account of her age.

Fortunately, such a pattern of drug prescribing is a caricature, but even in hospitals where close attention is given to minimising overtreatment in old age, polypharmacy remains a problem. In one review of psychiatric, geriatric, medical, and surgical wards it was found that patients were, on average, on 3.3 different drugs and that one-seventh were on six or more agents. Adding to the complexity of treatment was the fact that several drugs which could have been given once daily were given several times a day. Figure 2.3 illustrates this by showing that only a minority of patients received tricyclic antidepressants once daily.

Differences in disease patterns between old people in hospital and those living at home make it difficult to compare prescribing patterns within the two groups. In a group of patients over 75 treated in a practice, however, 87% were on at least one medication and 3.4% were on three or four drugs (Fig. 2.4). This

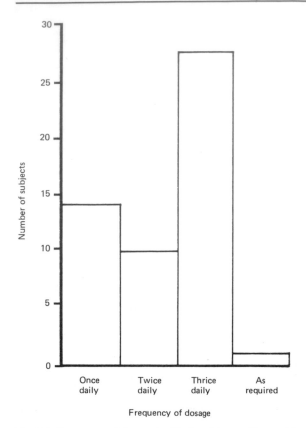

Fig. 2.3. Frequency of dosage in elderly subjects taking antidepressants (Christopher et al. 1978).

suggests that in the very old, polypharmacy is as great a problem in the community as in hospital.

Adverse Reactions

A reason for avoiding polypharmacy is that as the number of drugs used increases, so does the risk of drug side-effects. The risk is compounded in the elderly since, with increasing age, there is a striking rise in the incidence of side-effects (Fig. 2.5). A good example of the effects of ageing relate to benzodiazepine medication. Under the age of 40 the incidence of severe drowsiness is only 4.4% increasing to 10.9% in subjects over 70.

In a review of patients admitted to geriatric units in the United Kingdom, Williamson (1978) reported that between 2% and 3% of them had side-effects related to diuretics, major tranquillisers, antidepressants, and digitalis; between 1% and 2% had problems related to hypnotics, anticonvulsants, or analgesics;

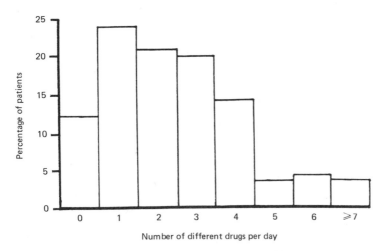

Fig. 2.4. Proportion of patients related to number of different drugs taken each day (Law and Chalmers 1976).

and 0.5%–1% had adverse reactions to hypotensives or rigidity controllers. A rather different picture emerged when he related side-effects to the number of patients on a particular drug. Here, just over 10% of patients who were on major tranquillisers, antidepressants, digitalis, hypotensives, or rigidity controllers had side-effects. This compared with only 5%–10% of those on diuretics or hypnotics, and less than 5% of those on analgesics. An indication of the practical importance of such adverse reactions is that in around 10% of men

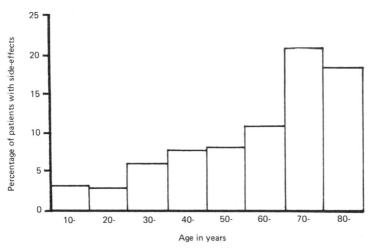

Fig. 2.5. Percentage of patients with drug side-effects related to age (Hurwitz 1969).

and women, admission to hospital was partially or wholly attributable to one of these. This compares with a figure of only 2.9% for patients of all ages who were admitted to hospital because of drug toxicity.

Reasons for the high incidence of adverse drug reactions in old age include changes in the first-pass metabolism, body distribution, plasma binding, renal excretion, hepatic metabolism, and tissue or organ sensitivity to drugs (Chap. 1). The situation is even more complex than this in that multiple pathology probably is an even more important factor than ageing in determining the way in which an elderly patient handles and responds to a drug. Thus, tables of dosage which relate simply to age, sex, and weight, though useful in children, are of little assistance in the elderly.

A better approach is simply to start off with a very low dose, and to increase this progressively until the desired effect is achieved. Drugs for which this applies include levodopa, phenothiazine tranquillisers, and beta-adrenoceptor blocking agents. In situations where a rapid effect is essential but where the drug has a high potential toxicity, regular blood concentrations may have to be measured. Examples here include gentamycin, cardiac glycosides, and anticon-

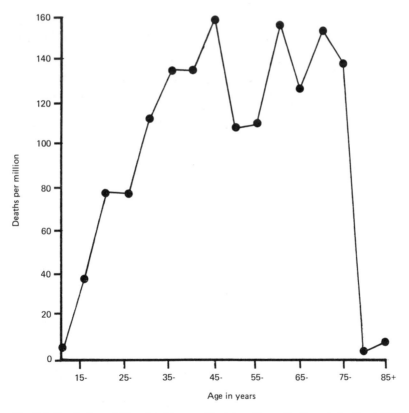

Fig. 2.6. Deaths by suicide related to age (Registrar General's Report, Scotland 1978).

vulsants. Drugs such as antidepressants pose a particular problem in that they are very toxic and their efficacy shows little relationship with doses or blood concentrations. Here the best approach is start off with small doses, rapidly increasing these, but monitoring closely for side-effects.

Self-poisoning

A particular form of drug poisoning which deserves special attention is that of intentional drug overdosage. Ageing is associated with a rising incidence of suicide (Fig. 2.6). The fall-off in extreme old age probably is related to the extreme frailty of people at risk. Figures on attempted suicide by drug overdosage are more difficult to come by, but it is likely that these mirror the pattern for suicide. In addition to being more frequent, overdosage in old age is more likely to result in death. This is because old people more often seek a permanent release from an intolerable situation. They are less likely to use overdosage as a "cry for help". Factors they may consider intolerable include bereavement, isolation, retirement, and poor physical health.

Added to this is the clear link between suicide or parasuicide and depression, a condition extremely common in the elderly. An example is that in one study 89% of people over 60 attempting suicide were suffering from a psychotic illness. In many instances such patients present to their doctors with hypochondriasis. If they are given potent drugs for this they may use them to end their lives. Even if depression is correctly identified, the administration of tricyclic or monoamine oxidase inhibitor antidepressants may put the patient at considerable risk. Prevention first involves identifying people at greatest risk (Table 2.2). Their problems can then either be treated or palliated.

Table 2.2. Elderly subjects at risk from suicide or parasuicide (Shulman 1978)

1. Elderly male
2. Mild to moderate depression with insomnia and physical symptoms
3. Isolation
4. Poor physical health
5. Recent bereavement
6. Recent previous suicide attempt
7. Access to means for suicide

Drug Interactions

Polypharmacy, apart from increasing the risk of drugs adversely affecting organs and tissues, makes it more likely that drugs will react with each other. A further factor is that the biological effects of ageing, such as impaired binding of drugs by albumin and decreased hepatic enzyme activity, further increase the likelihood of drug interactions.

Compliance

Even if a doctor keeps the number of drugs prescribed to a minimum, monitors patients for side-effects, and avoids prescribing drugs with major interactions, the problem remains that elderly patients may not take the drugs or, even worse, take the wrong drugs at the wrong time and in the wrong dosage.

There are a variety of explanations for poor compliance in old age. The most important is mental impairment. Healthy old people have little deterioration in mental function, other than some inability to process recent information and adapt to new situations. They usually compensate for this by using their long experience. Thus it is that they respond well to tasks relying upon educational attainment and linguistic ability, but are less at home in novel situations involving problem solving.

Such changes only have a marginal effect on their ability to take drugs. Indeed, prolonged training and fewer other demands on their memory may mean that they are more methodical and diligent. This, coupled with accentuated and unquestioning respect for authority, means that they often are more compliant than young patients. Such high compliance carries its own dangers since, in some instances, the only way in which patients avoid toxic effects is poor compliance and scepticism towards medical advice.

Unfortunately, old people most likely to be on medication are those most likely also to be suffering from some degree of mental impairment. The prevalence of severe mental impairment is about 2% in patients aged 65–74, through 10% in those between 75 and 84, rising to 25% in those of 85 and over. Patients with this have gross memory defects and behavioural abnormalities, so that a reasonable level of drug compliance is unlikely.

Physical handicap, though less important, also may pose problems. A partially sighted old lady has difficulty in identifying tablets, in reading labels on bottles, or in drawing up the correct dose of insulin. Likewise, a patient with Parkinsonism or arthritic hands may find that the lids on "child-proof" containers are also "granny-proof". She also has difficulty in opening tear-off bubble packs.

An early study on drug compliance by the elderly was conducted at the General Medical Clinic of the New York Hospital. Detailed questioning of 178 out-patients over the age of 60 revealed that 59% had made at least one mistake in medication, and that in this group many were making multiple errors (Fig. 2.7). While many mistakes were of little relevance, one quarter of the total made errors judged as being potentially serious.

Errors took a variety of forms (Table 2.3). The most common was omission. This often happened because patients had misunderstood their doctor's instructions, but in other instances lack of money or inability to get to a pharmacist because of disability were important. Another common problem was inaccurate information about the purpose and function of tablets, e.g. mistaking sleeping tablets for heart ones. Other patients increased dosage without seeking medical advice or, indeed, took medicines prescribed for their spouse. A few took drugs at the wrong time or in the wrong order. This often was related to inability to read labels or containers, or confusion about instructions given by the doctor.

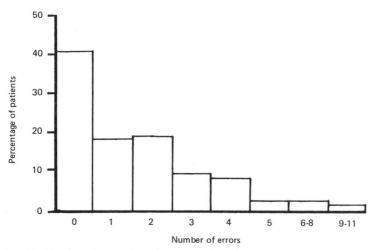

Fig. 2.7. Number of errors in medication made by out-patients aged over 60 years (Schwartz et al. 1962).

Patients making errors showed certain characteristics. Thus, those aged 75 years and over were more likely to make mistakes than those between 60 and 74 years. Again, those who were widowed, divorced, or separated were at greater risk than those who were single or married. Isolation and educational attainment also seemed to be important. Surprisingly, visual impairment had little effect on compliance, but ill health was important in that patients with five or more diagnoses were far more likely to make mistakes. Contrary to some other studies, there was no link between mistakes and the number of different tablets taken by an individual.

Compliance also was measured in elderly patients visited at a time of crisis by a geriatric physician at the request of a general practitioner. This again emphasised the importance of effective supervision for avoiding omissions in disabled old people (Table 2.4).

Table 2.3 Types of error made by out-patients aged over 60 years (Schwartz et al. 1962)

Type of error		Number
Omission		126
Self-medication		47
Incorrect dosage		26
Improper timing sequence		15
Inaccurate knowledge		55
	Total	269

Table 2.4. Proportion of patients omitting drugs at the time
of a geriatric assessment visit (Gibson and O'Hare 1968)

Category of patient	
Living alone unable to care for self	23%
Living alone able to care for self	29%
Living with people able to supervise	10%
Living with people unfit to supervise	35%

Self-medication often poses particular difficulties at the time of discharge
from hospital, when responsibility is transferred from the nursing staff to the
patient himself. Parkin et al. (1976) found that of 130 middle aged or elderly
patients discharged from general medical wards, 66 failed to follow their
prescribed drug regimen. Forty-six of these misunderstood the instructions,
while another 20 simply did not follow them. The proportion of errors increased
with the number of different drugs (Fig. 2.8) and with the number of daily doses
of a single drug prescribed (Fig. 2.9). A further problem was that patients, at
home, often took drugs prescribed before their admission to hospital.

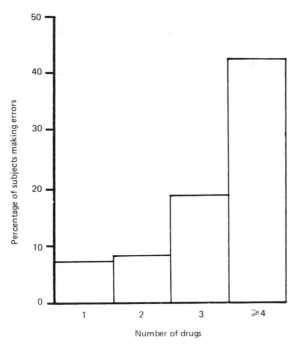

Fig. 2.8. Proportions of subjects making errors related to number of different drugs prescribed
(Parkin et al. 1976).

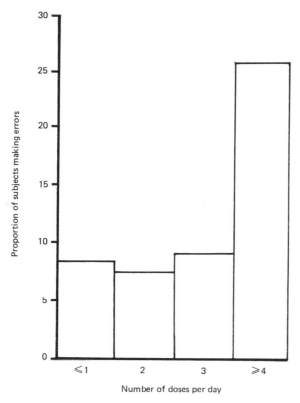

Fig. 2.9. Proportion of patients making errors in medication related to number of daily doses of individual drugs (Parkin et al. 1976).

Patients about to be discharged from a geriatric unit have even greater difficulties with medication. Many are vague about what tablets to take and when to take them; have difficulty in getting to their chemist or family doctor for prescriptions; and are unable to read labels on bottles. Most can open screw-top bottles and ordinary containers, but the majority have difficulty with child-proof containers. An area of particular confusion is recognising the stage at which the family doctor should be called in to take over prescribing from the hospital. This problem is compounded if communication is poor between hospital and general practitioner.

The pattern of limited compliance in patients admitted or discharged from hospital should not be transposed to old people in general living at home. An example is that, in a group practice, 75% of patients aged 75 years and over were able to repeat accurately the instructions for taking their medicines without first reading labels. This was found despite the fact that 17 labels were illegible, 4.5% of containers omitted to give the name of the drug and, in some instances, instructions were vague and non-specific, e.g. "two tablets as required". The only major problem was that 33% of patients left tablets in an exposed position, while many were unaware of how to dispose of tablets, so that younger members of the family were at increased risk. A reason for the small proportion of patients with compliance problems is that even over the age of 75, only a minority of patients suffer from severe physical or mental impairment. The remainder function as well as younger adults in adhering to instructions. If, then, scarce and expensive resources are to be used to improve compliance they should be directed to old people at risk, namely those living alone who also have mental impairment, depression, arthritis or paralysed hands, swallowing difficulties, limited mobility, or restricted vision.

Studies on drug compliance by the elderly have given rise to a large number of recommendations. The first is that the regime should be as simple as possible. Even young adults rarely take more than three different medicines per day correctly. Whenever feasible, three should be set as the upper limit for different preparations. Intermittent treatment also should be avoided. The instruction to take digoxin once daily 5 days a week almost certainly will cause trouble.

Directions should be as clear as possible so that it is essential that the container label should be legible by having large typed letters and figures. The name of the drug should always be given and this should be the official rather than the proprietary one. A switch from a formulation with one name to one with another may be very confusing. Instructions also should be specific as to dosage and timing. "Take three times per day after meals" is better than "Take as directed".

Compliance can also be improved by giving written or typed instructions separate from the label on the container. In one form this is a calendar with tear off sheets for each date and day of the week which gives the timing, the dose, the name and the purpose (e.g. "water tablet" for frusemide) of each medicine. An alternative is to provide a single card to which a sample of each drug is attached by adhesive tape. Against each sample is listed the name, the purpose, the dose and the timing of each drug (Fig. 2.10.). At a simpler level, a card with legible writing detailing the name, the purpose, the dose, and the timing of each drug is useful.

The design of the container also is important. Ability to identify a tablet usually is more important than shelf life, so that bottles should be made of clear rather than smoked material. A hand-sized container is better than a smaller

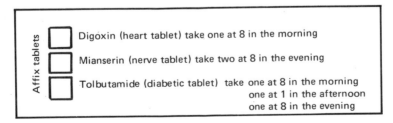

Fig. 2.10. Drug instructions to patient.

one, and it should have a screw or a clip top. Bottles with child-proof tops are inaccessible to old people with mental impairment, arthritic hands, or poor vision. Patients with arthritis also find problems with drugs in plastic bubble caps.

Much ingenuity has gone into devising automatic dispensers which will deliver drugs in the right dose at the right time. The Dosett box is such a system (Fig. 2.11). It is a plastic container with seven parallel compartments for each day of the week. Each of these is divided into four sub-compartments representing four time periods of the day. Seven transparent slides cover the compartments. When these are slid down they uncover in turn sub-compartments 1, 2, 3, and 4. The box is loaded with tablets in the appropriate compartments each week and is then used by the patient. The days and times are printed clearly with raised lettering, and boxes in braille are available for patients who are completely blind. A criticism of such a system is that its very ingenuity means that patients require a modicum of intelligence and considerable training. Certainly, in one study, the use of the box seemed to have no advantage over a simple programme of training in improving compliance.

Pharmacists have given thought to producing personal bubble packs for patients in which drugs for a particular day are packaged in the one section. Dating the section and marking the day of the week would allow the patient to see whether or not he was keeping up to date with his medication. A limitation of the system is that patients with weak or arthritic hands have difficulty in opening packs. A more fundamental problem is that if a patient does not have the mental capacity to follow a drug regime using labels on bottles assisted, perhaps, with a drug identification card, he is unlikely to cope with a dispenser or calendar pack.

Attention must be directed also to the formulation of medicines. Some old people prefer liquids to pills so that many of the more widely used agents are available in both syrup and liquid form. The taste of a drug may be critical, and can sometimes be modified by mixing it with an appropriate drink. Manufacturers even may have to consider the colour of tablets. Patients consider that green tablets are good for phobias, white ones useful in muscle tension, and red ones ideal for rheumatism. Again, triangular tablets are more likely to improve concentration than round ones. Such seemingly trivial preferences have major consequences outside the scientific confines of a hospital ward.

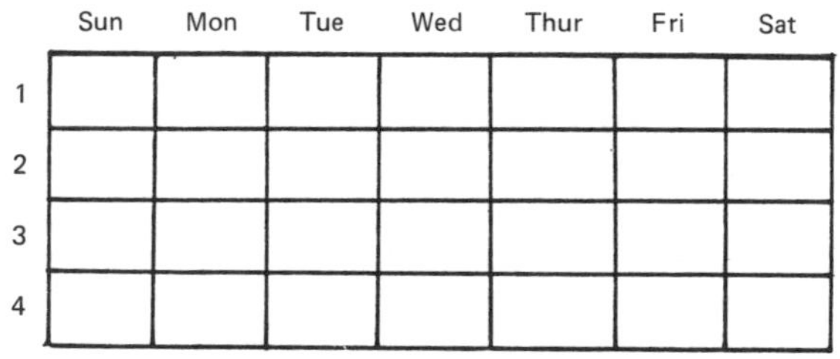

	Sun	Mon	Tue	Wed	Thur	Fri	Sat
1							
2							
3							
4							

Fig. 2.11. Principle of the Dosett box.

Particular attention should be given to compliance at the time that the patient is discharged home from hospital. In a pre-discharge programme at Glasgow, the consultant first simplifies the drug regime as far as possible (Boxendale et al. 1978). A pharmacist then reviews with the patient the most suitable form of labels and containers; going on to show him each medicine and explain its function. He then issues a card providing details about drugs, times, and dosages. The patient is then given 2 days' supply of drugs and is encouraged to keep them in his locker and to take them at times which will be convenient after he goes home. After 2 days the pharmacist checks, by discussion and observation, on whether or not the drugs have been taken appropriately. He then gives a further drug supply and continues the process until the patient is deemed ready for discharge. Drug dispensers can be incorporated into the training programme, but there is little evidence that they have much overall effect on compliance.

Nursing staff often are worried about hospital patients taking their own tablets. Issues such as the dangers of hoarding, of theft by demented patients, or of who is responsible for overdosages loom large. It should be recognised, however, that such problems are likely to be even greater after discharge. A well documented and researched policy on pre-discharge self-administration of drugs should resolve most medico-legal objections.

At discharge, it is important that the general practitioner should know not only what drugs a patient is on, but what formulations are being used. Changes in the size, colour, or shape of tablets may be very disturbing, so that the general practitioner should devise a system which ensures that the patient gets a continuing supply of the appropriate drug. It also is useful if a district nurse or health visitor can visit at an early stage to ensure that drugs no longer being used are discarded. Advice on keeping potentially lethal agents out of the grasp of children also is important.

Some patients fail to measure up to the demands of self-medication. If the patient lives alone the question of discharge should be reconsidered. It may even be necessary to arrange admission to a residential home. The patient may be fortunate in having a relative who can supervise treatment, but some relatives are frail and befuddled themselves. Time should be spent, therefore, ensuring that the relative really does know details of the timing, dosage, and function of the drugs.

Once the patient is settled again at home, the general practitioner has to consider how best to monitor drug treatment. Old people are unlikely to refer themselves. Indeed, in one practice half the elderly patients on long-term treatment had not been in contact with their doctor over the previous 6 months. It is impossible to visit regularly every old person on drugs, so that attention should be directed to high-risk groups. These include people living alone, those with severe mental or physical impairment, and the very old, i.e. those over 85. If she has enough time, the health visitor often is the best person to keep such people under review. Obviously she cannot supervise day-to-day medication, but she can alert the doctor to the individual whose poor compliance may be life-threatening.

A potential source of confusion is the day hospital, where patients are under the surveillance of both general practitioner and hospital doctor. One way of tackling the problem is for the hospital doctor and general practitioner to contact each other by phone. An alternative is for both to fill in the same card listing medication. This, if well designed, can have the added advantage of providing the patient with information on the timing, dosage, and function of his medication.

Self-medication

An important aspect of therapeutics often forgotten by health care professionals is the use of drugs purchased by patients direct from pharmacists. In one general practice, almost half of the patients over the age of 75 regularly used medicine obtained in this way. Preparations most commonly purchased are analgesics and laxatives. Interestingly, although there is a marked increase in the number of people on prescribed drugs, the proportion on non-prescribed ones remains remarkably stationary throughout adult life (Fig. 2.12). This

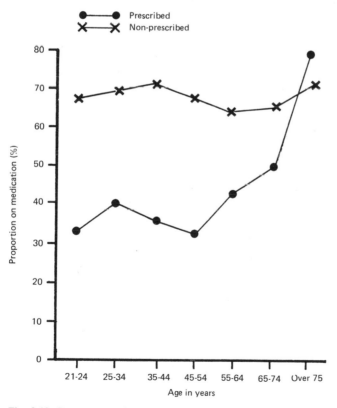

Fig. 2.12. Percentages of subjects on prescribed and non-prescribed medication related to age (Dunnell and Cartwright 1972).

might represent a more stoical approach to minor symptoms in old age, but it is more likely that old people often are unable to afford the cost of non-prescribed medication.

The direct availability of drugs from the pharmacist without recourse to a doctor probably saves the health service a great deal in terms of man-hours and money. Thus, while 70% of people with a headache take medication, only one in 200 visits a general practitioner (Table 2.5). Balanced against this saving are the hazards of self-medication. Drugs may be taken for the wrong reason, e.g. aspirin to relieve dyspepsia; the same ingredient may be taken in several different preparations for the same symptom; an agent may interact with drugs prescribed by the doctor or vice versa; too large a dose may be taken; and drugs may be altered by inappropriate storage.

Table 2.5. Symptoms recorded in women related to medication taken and visit to general practitioner (Morrell 1979)

Symptom	Proportion taking medication	Proportion visiting general practitioner
Headache	70%	0.5%
Backache	38%	0.9%
Abdominal pain	53%	2.6%
Sore throat	59%	3.0%
Cough	78%	3.2%

Some of these problems might be avoided if patients followed rules developed by a working group of the Council of Europe. These are: to take care of all medicines; to read directions carefully; never to treat a symptom for more than a week without consulting a doctor; to consult a doctor if a drug fails to have the desired effect; if already on drugs prescribed by a doctor to consult him before taking a non-prescribed agent; to keep drugs in a dark, cool place away from children; to get rid of medicine kept for longer than a year; and to *destroy completely* any unused medicine. Whether a health education programme will be effective in persuading old people to follow these recommendations remains to be seen.

References

Boxendale C, Gourlay M, Gibson IIJM (1978) A self-medication retraining programme. Br Med J 2: 1278–1279

Christopher LJ, Ballinger BR, Shepherd AMM, Ramsay A, Crooks J (1978) Drug prescribing patterns in the elderly: a cross sectional study of inpatients. Age Ageing 7: 74–82

Hall MRP (1973) Drug therapy in the elderly. Br Med J 3: 582–584

Hurwitz N (1969) Predisposing factors in adverse reactions to drugs. Br Med J 1: 536–540
Law R, Chalmers C (1976) Medicines and elderly people: a general practice survey. Br Med J 1: 565–566
Morrell DC (1979) Facts and issues in self care. In: Anderson JAD (ed) Self medication, MTP, Lancaster, pp 19–30
Parkin DM, Henney CR, Quirk J, Crooks J (1976) Deviation from prescribed treatment after discharge from hospital. Br Med J 2: 686–688
Schwartz D, Wang M, Zeity L, Goss J (1962) Medication errors made by elderly, chronically ill patients. Am J Public Health 52: 2018–2029
Shulman K (1978) Suicide and parasuicide in old ages a review. Age Ageing 7: 201–209
Williamson J (1978) Prescribing problems in the elderly. Practitioner 220: 749–758
Wilson LA, Lawson IR, Brass W (1962) Multiple disorders in the elderly. A clinical and statistical study. Lancet 2: 841–843

3 Disorders of the Heart

Congestive Cardiac Failure

Congestive cardiac failure is extremely common in old age, ankle oedema occurring in 22% of patients between 70 and 75 in general practice, and accounting for the fact that in those over 75, 18% are on diuretics, and 17% on digoxin (Currie et al. 1974; Law and Chalmers 1976). Treatment of the disorder does not differ qualitatively from that in younger individuals. However, changes in the renal function and in the electrolyte and metabolic status of old people modify their response to cardiac glycosides and diuretics, and increase the risk of side-effects.

Cardiac Glycosides

Rationale for Use

Doubts about efficacy of cardiac glycosides, their narrow therapeutic index, and the serious effect which renal impairment has on their duration of action, have led to a critical reappraisal of their usefulness in the elderly. Most authorities are agreed on their value in controlling the heart rate in atrial fibrillation. A possible exception in the elderly is atrial fibrillation associated with incomplete atrioventricular block.

There is greater doubt as to their efficacy in congestive cardiac failure accompanied by a sinus rhythm. MacHaffie and his colleagues demonstrated that if digoxin was given to patients in sinus rhythm who had congestive cardiac failure controlled with diuretics, it had no effect on symptoms, heart rate, respiratory rate, ventilation and respiration quotients, or workload achieved. In another series, Dall (1981) reported that digoxin was withdrawn without detriment from 59 out of 80 elderly patients. There is the possibility, however, that the reason that digoxin often can be withdrawn successfully is that blood levels of the glycoside often are submaximal and thus unlikely to be benefiting the patient. Again some patients on digoxin may not have been suffering from congestive cardiac failure in the first place.

There remains, however, a small subgroup of patients in sinus rhythm who deteriorate when digoxin is stopped. Most commonly this happens when their heart rhythm changes to atrial fibrillation, but occasionally there is deterioration in ventricular function.

The reason why not all patients respond to glycosides is not clear. It may be that a high sympathetic tone blocks their action. In such a situation a peripheral vasodilator might be useful. Whatever the theory for the efficacy of digoxin, the practical approach is that patients with sinus rhythm in congestive cardiac failure should first be treated with a diuretic. If this does not work the dose of diuretic should be increased, and if this still does not work digoxin should be added. If over the course of several months the condition of the patient stabilises, the cardiotropic effect of digoxin may decline. It is important, therefore, to review patients regularly and consider withdrawing the glycoside.

Administration

An age-related decline in the glomerular filtration rates means that old people excrete less digoxin, and require lower loading and maintenance doses than young adults. Usually the loading dose is 0.5–0.75 mg. The maintenance dose is more difficult to determine, being dependent on a large number of variables including sex, age, weight, mobility, heart rhythm, serum creatinine concentrations, whether or not the patient is on diuretics, and whether or not he is an in-patient. The relevance of being in hospital is that such patients tend to have more severe muscle wasting, more severe heart failure, and a lower fat intake. A variety of nomograms and weighting scales have been devised by clinicians so that dosage can be determined on the basis of sex, age, weight, and renal function.

Many others use the simple rule of thumb whereby they give 0.25 mg daily to an elderly patient of average build with a normal blood urea. If he is emaciated or has marginal elevation of his blood urea a dose of 0.125 mg daily is more appropriate. Where there is gross renal impairment a dose of 0.0625 mg often will be adequate.

Where less care is taken in calculating the dose of digoxin, more care has to be taken in monitoring its effect. In youth toxicity usually is heralded by anorexia or nausea, but these symptoms often are absent in old age. A close watch must be kept, therefore, on the pulse rate. A drop to less than 60 beats per minute should lead to an urgent review of treatment. Usually bradycardia precedes the onset of arrhythmias, but this is not always the case, so that a regular check has to be kept on not only the rate but also the rhythm of the pulse. At the opposite extreme, the dose may be too small. This often is the case where too much emphasis is placed on impaired renal function and a dose of only 0.0625 mg daily given. Here a failure to reduce the pulse rate often is the clue that something is wrong.

Though inadequate dosage is an important reason for an inadequate response other factors deserve consideration. There is the evidence, already presented, that where there is sinus rhythm, digoxin has relatively little effect on cardiac contractility, and that this tends to wear off with continued use. Again, compliance may be a problem. Johnston et al. (1978) found that 36% of patients admitted to hospital had been taking less than the prescribed dose of digoxin, and that another 14% had been taking more than this. In general practice the situation was similar in that around half of patients were non-compliant, about one in 20 not taking any digoxin at all. In ensuring compliance it is important to avoid complex regimes. There is no reason why digoxin should not be given once rather than several times a day. Again, schedules prescribing doses every second day or 5 days a week should be avoided.

The efficacy of digoxin also is dependent on the plasma calcium concentration. Calcium plays an important part in myocardial contractility, so that patients with hypocalcaemia may be resistant to the effects of digoxin. In old age, where vitamin D deficiency is common, this may be much more important that is currently recognised.

The most accurate way of determining the adequacy or otherwise of a dose of digoxin is to measure its plasma concentration. The therapeutic range is 1.0–2.6 mmol/l. An assay is particularly useful if there has been a poor clinical response to digoxin. Subtherapeutic concentrations indicate too small a dose or, more frequently in sick old people, poor compliance. The assay is equally useful in confirming that less typical side-effects such as confusion are related to digoxin overdosage rather than a coincidental illness.

Side-effects

As in youth, cardiotoxic effects of cardiac glycosides in old age include pulsus bigeminus, multiple ventricular or supraventricular extra-systoles, ventricular and supraventricular tachycardias, all degrees of heart block, and ventricular fibrillation with sudden death. The high rate of cardiotoxicity in old people on digoxin relates to their impaired renal function. Another factor may be increased myocardial sensitivity due to potassium depletion often resulting from diuretic therapy. Here, the critical factor probably is a low ratio of extra- to intracellular potassium. Concern over the possibility of a low total body or total exchangeable potassium level in the face of a normal serum potassium concentration probably is unwarranted.

Cardiac glycosides also may interfere with cerebral function and, in old age, this may manifest itself as an acute confusional state. This often precedes cardiac signs of toxicity and there is clear evidence that it is related to the effects of digoxin rather than the anoxia of heart failure, or dehydration and electrolyte depletion due to diuretic therapy. In individuals however it can be difficult to distinguish digoxin toxicity from the myriad other causes of acute and chronic mental impairment. A long history of mental impairment and clinical or biochemical evidence for a physical cause of confusion makes the latter more likely. If doubt remains, a plasma digoxin concentration may clinch the diagnosis. Obviously, if confusion is due to digoxin toxicity, the drug must be stopped. There may then be a delay of up to 2 weeks before the mental state improves. The biochemical basis for this bizarre side-effect has not been identified.

Diuretics

Cardiac Failure

As in young patients, a diuretic is the drug of first choice for the management of congestive cardiac failure in the elderly. Since metabolic homoeostasis usually is impaired, cardiac failure should be corrected as gently as possible. Too rapid a loss of fluid and electrolytes is likely to cause uraemia, hypotension, collapse, and mental confusion. Thiazide diuretics should be used, therefore, whenever possible.

If the cardiac failure is acute or if it fails to respond to thiazides a short-acting "loop" diuretic should be introduced. Those used most widely are bumetanide and frusemide. Both have a wide dose/response curve so that they can be increased progressively until an adequate diuresis is obtained. Bumetanide has a shorter duration of action than frusemide. This has advantages if it is decided to increase fluid loss by giving a diuretic twice daily. The short duration of action means that, even if it is given in the early evening, it is unlikely to cause nocturnal incontinence.

Once a short-acting diuretic has stabilised cardiac failure, consideration should be given to either reducing the dose or switching back to a thiazide diuretic. While this is being done, however, the patient should be monitored closely for signs of fluid retention. In hospital the simplest way of doing this is to weigh him daily. At home, reliance has to be placed on looking at the neck veins and listening to the lung bases.

Idiopathic Oedema

In many old people oedema is confined to the lower limbs. This usually is the result of prolonged immobility in which there is a failure of muscle pump activity. A high incidence of subclinical deep leg thrombosis may also be important. Local treatment involves applying elastic stockings or one way stretch bandages. Though elastic stockings are easier to put on they often exert insufficient pressure, so that bandaging is preferable. Crepe bandages are not stiff enough and are completely useless. To avoid oedema of the distal foot the bandage must be applied from the toes upwards.

Diuretics are of limited value in that the oedema is not accompanied by an increased plasma volume. They merely make the patient dehydrated. This can be prevented if fluid is allowed to return to the vascular compartment by elevating the lower limbs before giving a diuretic. This, however, interferes with rehabilitation. A solution might be to give a diuretic with a very short duration of action, such as bumetanide. The patient could then go to bed in the late afternoon or early evening and take the drug at the same time as this.

Inappropriate Treatment

Diuretics often are given when oedema due to immobility is mistaken for congestive cardiac failure. Again the cause of the oedema often resolves. It is important, therefore, to review regularly the need for diuretics in old people. In a study by Burr and colleagues in one geriatric unit only 33 of 141 patients on diuretics were judged to require them (Burr et al. 1977). When 54 of the 108 remaining were changed from diuretic to placebo, only eight of them developed substantial fluid retention. Diuretics, therefore, often can be stopped in old people, but while this is being done, it is important to keep a close watch for fluid retention.

Side-effects

Salt and Water Depletion.   Age-related changes in renal function mean that though, under baseline conditions, old people are able to maintain a satisfactory fluid and electrolyte balance, even a minor change in intake or output is likely to cause severe derangement.

An example is that sodium depletion usually causes an increased renal excretion of water so that there is no change in the serum sodium concentration. Once the extra-cellular volume falls below a critical level, however, the mechanism ceases to work, so that there is fluid retention accompanied by hyponatraemia. Even minor renal impairment enhances this effect, so that diuretic-induced hyponatraemia is particularly common in the elderly. Large doses of isotonic saline are required to correct the imbalance. This can be advocated in young patients who usually cope if salt replacement is over-enthusiastic. In old age, however, homoeostasis is less effective and such treatment may cause salt and water overload. A less dramatic, but safer response is to stop the diuretic and to wait for the hyponatraemia to correct itself.

Congestive cardiac failure itself may cause hyponatraemia. A popular explanation is that hypoxaemia interferes with the ability of the cell membrane to pump in potassium and pump out sodium. An alternative may be that there is an expansion of the extra-cellular fluid volume due to (1) a reduced renal plasma flow rate, which reduces the volume of urine reaching the renal tubules; (2) a low effective intra-arterial volume stimulating antidiuretic hormone secretion; or (3) anoxia interfering with the response of osmoreceptors to hyponatraemia. In this condition, treatment should be directed at correcting the underlying disorder. The oral or parenteral administration of salt may be disastrous.

Potassium Depletion.   There is no doubt that thiazide diuretics cause a rapid and persistent fall in the serum potassium concentration. "Loop" diuretics are implicated less frequently. It should be noted, however, that in one surveillance programme, 3.6% of patients on frusemide developed hypokalaemia (Green-blatt et al. 1977). Old people may be at particular risk in that their reduced fat-free mass means that they have reduced intracellular reserves of potassium. Their dietary intakes of potassium also are often deficient.

Over the last 10 years, it has emerged that there is often little relationship between serum concentrations and total quantities of potassium in the body. There is controversy as to whether diuretics really cause potassium depletion. In young and middle-aged adults certainly, diuretics seem to have little effect on total body potassium status. Elderly patients with reduced potassium reserves are at greater risk of depletion by diuretics.

Another controversial issue is that a reduction in the ratio of extra- to intracellular potassium probably has greater effect on cardiac and skeletal muscle function than an absolute reduction in intracellular potassium. It may be that the debate has revolved a full circle and that physicians should be paying greater regard to serum potassium concentrations rather than measures of total potassium status. Such a change in approach would greatly simplify many clinical decisions.

The most important effect of potassium depletion is that it compromises cardiac function. Electrocardiographic effects of this include prolonged PR and QT intervals, low T waves, U waves, and a depressed ST segment. These may be accompanied by a wide range of conduction defects and arrhythmias. This is particularly troublesome if a cardiac glycoside is being used. In old people, potassium depletion also may interfere with regulation of the peripheral circulation and cause postural hypotension.

There is little doubt that potassium depletion associated with hypokalaemia and a low extra- to intracellular potassium ratio is accompanied by skeletal muscle weakness. It is less clear whether milder degrees of potassium depletion cause weakness. People with low potassium intakes have been reported to have a reduced grip strength even when the serum potassium was normal. Conversely, low red cell potassium concentrations may not be associated with muscle weakness.

There is uncertainty also about the effect of potassium depletion on mental function. Potassium supplements have been reported to alleviate depression and improve mental function in old people with dietary deficiency. Certainly elderly patients with depression have low total exchangeable potassium levels. However, this probably is a reflection of potassium levels being pushed down by corticosteroid hyperactivity induced by stress. In dementia low total exchangeable levels of potassium are the result of cell loss, and the ratio of potassium to dry body weight actually is increased. It is unlikely then that potassium depletion is a major treatable cause of either depression or dementia.

The fundamental question which all these observations raise is whether it is safe to treat old people with a diuretic alone. If the patient is on a cardiac glycoside, the risks of cardiotoxicity are unacceptably high. In other situations the need for adjuvant treatment is less clear and it is reasonable to give a diuretic alone so long as the serum potassium concentration is monitored regularly.

Potassium depletion can be treated with either potassium supplements or potassium-sparing diuretics. In elderly patients with congestive cardiac failure, supplements have little effect on the total body potassium status. They are more effective at increasing low serum potassium concentrations but, even here, large doses are required. The minimal dose required to prevent hypokalaemia in sick elderly patients on diuretics is 24 mmol daily. Table 3.1 lists the amounts of

Table 3.1. Potassium supplements

Preparation	Potassium content per tablet
Kloref	6.7 mmol
Sando K	12.0 mmol (only 8 mmol Cl⁻)
Slow K	8.0 mmol

potassium in various preparations. It is important that the potassium cation be balanced by chloride anion.

Apart from increasing the risk of hyperkalaemia, potassium salts are highly irritant. Old people who fail to swallow tablets often develop mouth ulcers. They also have impaired oesophageal motility, so that they are more likely to suffer from oesophageal ulceration and stenosis. Fortunately, there have been few reported cases of this.

The most commonly used potassium-sparing agents are spironolactone, triamterine, and amiloride, either given alone or in combination with a thiazide diuretic. Apparent differences in the efficacy of these agents probably reflect differences in the extent to which they have been investigated. All are effective in correcting hypokalaemia. Unfortunately, their efficacy cannot always be predicted. Sometimes they do not correct hypokalaemia, and on other occasions they are too potent, causing hyperkalaemia.

In terms of efficacy, there probably is not much to choose between supplements and sparing agents. A major advantage for sparing agents is that both in terms of taste and size they are more palatable. Compliance thus is more likely. This can be guaranteed where both diuretic and sparing agent are combined in one tablet. Combinations of diuretic and supplement also are available, but the quantities of potassium contained in these may not match up to the needs of the elderly patient.

Calcium and Magnesium Imbalance

Thiazide diuretics reduce the renal excretion of calcium to cause a mild hypercalcaemia. There is evidence that in the elderly at least hypercalcaemia may be as important as hypokalaemia in accentuating the cardiotoxic effects of glycosides. If this is confirmed it may prove important to monitor serum calcium as well as serum potassium concentrations in patients receiving thiazide diuretics.

Most diuretics may be responsible for magnesium depletion. Clinical symptoms of this include depression, ataxia, muscular weakness, gastro-intestinal disorders, and increased cardiac sensitivity to glycosides. Old people on diuretics often have hypomagnesaemia. It remains to be seen whether this is responsible for the numerous symptoms found in old people and whether magnesium supplements will resolve these.

Carbohydrate Intolerance

The effects which both ageing and diuretics have on carbohydrate metabolism mean that old people on diuretics are at particular risk of developing diabetes mellitus. In one large-scale trial involving a thiazide and a potassium-sparing diuretic, there was, over 2 years, an appreciable rise in fasting blood glucose concentrations, and a deterioration in glucose tolerance. It is not clear whether these changes led to an increased incidence of ketoacidosis or other complications of diabetes.

Hyperuricaemia

Old people often have high serum concentrations or uric acid and diuretic therapy produces further elevation. However, there are few reports of diuretics precipitating gout in old people. Concern should be reserved for patients with a family history or previous episodes of gout.

Incontinence

Doctors often are faced with the dilemma of removing excess fluid from a patient in whom cerebrovascular disease, a lax pelvic floor, or an enlarged prostate is already causing urinary frequency. The problem is compounded if, in addition, mobility is restricted by locomotor or neurological disease. The first essential is for the ward staff to record accurately episodes of micturition and urinary incontinence. It then may be possible to tailor diuretic therapy to the requirements of a patient. If he is incontinent during the morning, a long-acting rather than a short-acting diuretic may be more appropriate. A short-acting diuretic may be more useful if the patient has nocturia and nocturnal incontinence.

Vasodilators

Traditionally, treatment of congestive cardiac failure has consisted of increasing the force of cardiac contraction and decreasing the volume of circulation. More recently, attention has been directed at decreasing resistance to cardiac outflow by dilating the peripheral arterial system. In addition, drugs relaxing venous smooth muscle have been used to enhance the effect of diuretics in lowering the central venous pressure.

Vasodilators have been used to great effect in patients with acute left ventricular failure. Sodium nitroprusside, phentolamine, glyceryl trinitrate, and salbutamol are given intravenously using an infusion pump. Dosage is modified in the light of changes in the systemic and in the capillary wedge pressures. Isosorbide dinitrate is given sublingually, but it still is necessary to monitor systemic and pulmonary pressure. Such treatment should only be undertaken by an experienced cardiologist in a centre with adequate delivery and monitoring equipment. Even with this, restraint should be used when dealing with the elderly. Vasodilation may "steal" blood away from stenosed vessels, so that the patient may recover from his failure at the expense of a stroke, decerebration, a mesenteric infarction, or peripheral gangrene.

Vasodilators also have a place in the management of chronic congestive cardiac failure refractory to glycosides and diuretics. Both hydralazine and prazosin, when given orally, are effective in increasing cardiac output in this situation. Captopril, an inhibitor of angiotensin conversion, also has been used to good effect in the management of glycoside and diuretic resistant heart failure. Limitations to the widespread use of these agents, particularly in the elderly, are that careful cardiological monitoring is necessary and that there is only a narrow margin between reducing peripheral resistance and causing either postural or generalised hypotension.

Coronary Artery Disease

Angina

In view of the high prevalence of electrocardiographic abnormalities, and of coronary artery atheroma demonstrable at autopsy, it is surprising that angina is not more common in the elderly. Factors which prevent this happening include an increase in the threshold for deep pain sensation; restriction of mobility by locomotor or neurological disorders; and angina present earlier in life resolving as a collateral coronary circulation develops.

The mainstay of treatment is sublingual glyceryl trinitrate, but old people with a tendency to postural hypotension and with impaired cerebral autoregulation are at increased risk of sustaining syncopal attacks following the peripheral vasodilator effect of the drug.

Attention must be directed to preventing as well as controlling attacks. Table 3.2 details some of the agents used for this purpose.

The drugs most widely used for this purpose are the beta-blocking agents. If short-acting ones such as oxprenolol or propranolol are to be effective they must be given several times a day. Thus, if there are compliance problems there may be an advantage in using long-acting agents such as atenolol or nadolol. The diminished first-pass metabolism of beta-blockers in old age means that smaller doses should be used than in youth or middle age.

Elderly patients with coincidental congestive cardiac failure should not be given a beta-blocker. It is better to use an alternative type of drug than to resort to a beta-blocker with intrinsic sympatheticomimetic activity or to one which is combined with a diuretic. Coronary artery disease often is accompanied by peripheral vascular disease, particularly in old age. This may well be exacerbated by the vasoconstrictor effect of a beta-blocker. Here again it is better to use an alternative anti-anginal agent than experiment with a cardio-selective beta-blocker.

Table 3.2. Drugs used to prevent episodes of angina

Drug	Dosage
A: Beta-blocking agents	
Propranolol	20–60 mg three times daily
Oxprenolol	40–120 mg twice daily
Atenolol	50 mg once daily
Nadolol	40–120 mg once daily
B: Nitrates	
Sustained-action glyceryl trinitrate	2.6–6.4 mg three times daily
Isosorbide dinitrate	5–20 mg four times daily
C: Calcium antagonists	
Nifedipine	10–20 mg three times daily

Note: Only examples of drugs in each category are given.

Nitrates with a sustained action are valuable alternatives to beta-blocking agents, particularly if the patient has congestive cardiac failure or peripheral vascular disease. They can be used either alone, or in combination with a beta-blocker. The latter approach, of course, smacks of polypharmacy and should only be used in the elderly where the maximum dose of a single agent has been ineffective. The main limitation to the use of nitrates in the elderly is their tendency to cause postural hypotension. There is also the disadvantage that their pharmocokinetics and pharmacodynamics are poorly understood, so that there is no information on whether their dosage should be modified in old age.

Another agent which controls angina by reducing peripheral arterial resistance is the calcium antagonist nifedipine. It may be particularly useful in elderly patients who also have congestive cardiac failure, in that it reduces peripheral resistance and thus increases cardiac output. Unfortunately, the drug also has a negative inotropic effect. Thus, if added to a beta-blocking agent, it sometimes precipitates cardiac failure. This is another reason why combinations of anti-anginal agents should be avoided in the elderly.

Myocardial Infarction

The first problem of treating myocardial infarction in old age is recognising the condition, because it often presents with atypical symptoms such as confusion, syncope, hemiparesis, or dizziness. This pattern might be partly a reflection on the type of patients referred to a geriatric unit. Nonetheless, it is important to review initially all patients presenting with vague symptoms if myocardial infarction is to be recognised and treated appropriately.

The question arises as to where an elderly patient with myocardial infarction should be treated. If he has severe mental and physical impairment, it is best to manage him symptomatically at home if adequate support from relatives is available. With this proviso, however, elderly patients with myocardial infarctions should be treated in the same way as their younger counterparts. Patients over the age of 70 admitted to a coronary care unit have a higher mortality and rate of complication, and stay longer in hospital than younger patients. Thus, if anything, the management of myocardial infarction is more difficult in old age. Argument remains as to the general efficacy of the coronary care unit, but if it is used at all, its services should not be denied to the elderly.

Old people with chest pain due to myocardial infarction should be given an opiate. However, the half-life of morphine is prolonged in old age. There also may be an increased tissue sensitivity to the drug. The result is that many elderly patients on opiates develop signs of toxicity. These include a reduced level of consciousness, and respiratory depression. The problem should be tackled by starting with small doses, and not giving these more often than eight-hourly.

Pulmonary congestion should be treated with oxygen and diuretics. Patients in shock may respond to vasodilators, but these should only be given when cardiac monitoring is feasible. The incidence of cardiac arrhythmias may be reduced by giving an intravenous bolus followed by an infusion of lignocaine. Beta-blocking agents also prevent arrhythmias, but their higher incidence of side-effects precludes their use in this situation.

After the acute episode, attention should be directed at preventing a recurrence of the myocardial infarction. Beta-blocking agents have the theoretical benefits of reducing the likelihood of arrhythmias and reducing myocardial metabolic requirements, thereby decreasing the size of a subsequent infarct. Both timolol and metoprolol reduce mortality if given as long-term treatment after a myocardial infarction, and are almost as effective in patients aged 65–74 as in younger groups (Norwegian Multicentre Study Group 1980; Hjalmarson et al. 1981).

The role of anticoagulants in reducing mortality after myocardial infarction has been investigated extensively. They may be of marginal value in young and middle-aged men, but are ineffective in elderly patients of either sex. Antiplatelet agents including sulphinpyrazone and aspirin also have been used in long-term prophylaxis after a myocardial infarction (Anturane Reinfarction Trial Research Group 1980). Sulphinpyrazone is of marginal benefit in the first 6 months after an infarction, but further studies are required to establish the value of aspirin. The ease with which these drugs can be given and their relative freedom from serious side-effects in the dosage suggested mean that they would have obvious attractions for prophylactic treatment in the elderly. More evidence on their efficacy, however, is required before their widespread use can be recommended, particularly in old people already on far too many drugs.

Cardiac Arrhythmias

The management of these disorders is essentially the same for any age group.

Infective Endocarditis

This condition, though common in middle-aged subjects, reaches a peak incidence in those aged 61–70 years. In older patients there is a steep fall in the incidence of recorded cases. This might represent both reduced diagnostic enthusiasm and a less clear-cut presentation, rather than a real reduction.

A prerequisite of effective treatment is accurate and early diagnosis. This is difficult in old people, in whom the condition often may mimic a psychiatric disturbance, renal failure, or gastro-intestinal malignancy. The only clues to the condition may be a cardiac murmur and a grossly elevated erythrocyte sedimentation rate.

The next essential is to identify accurately the infecting organism. At present the most common are staphylococci and streptococci. With increasing age a greater proportion of infections are associated with streptococci, reflecting possibly a lower incidence of both narcotic addiction and valve replacement in this group. Organisms less commonly responsible for endocarditis include *Escherichia, Haemophilus, Pseudomonas, Pneumococcus, Brucella, Candida,* and *Coxiella.* There also is a group of between 5% and 10% in whom blood culture is persistently negative.

The antibiotic regimen used depends on the nature of the organism (Table 3.3). A point of particular importance in the elderly is that a close watch should

Table 3.3. Antibiotic therapy in infective endocarditis (MacDonald 1979)

Organism		Antibiotic	Dose	Route
Strep. viridans		Penicillin	10–12 mega-units daily for 2 weeks	Continuous IV infusion
	then	Amoxycillin	1 g 6-hourly	Oral
Strep. faecalis		Penicillin	20 mega-units daily	Continuous IV infusion
	and	Streptomycin	Check blood levels	IM injections
	or	Gentamycin		IM injections
Staph. pyogenes		Flucloxacillin	0.5–1 g 4-hourly	IV injections
	or	Cephadrine	0.5–1 g 6-hourly	IV injections

(Other antibiotics including sodium fusidate, lincomycin, or vancomycin may be used where the sensitivity of the organism indicates.)

Gram-negative organisms		Amoxycillin	1 g 6-hourly	IV injections
	and	Gentamycin		IM injections

(Cephadrine or carbenicillin may be used in place of amoxycillin where the sensitivity of the organism indicates.)

Culture negative		Penicillin	20 mega-units daily	Continuous IV infusion
	and	Streptomycin	Check blood levels	IM injections
	or	Gentamycin		IM injections

be kept on streptomycin and gentamycin blood levels. Renal impairment and increased organ sensitivity increase the dangers of these drugs in old age. Again, if a cephalosporin is required, then a non-nephrotoxic form such as cephadrine or cefuroxime should be used. Whatever antibiotics are used it is essential that treatment be continued for at least 6 weeks.

In a frail elderly patient there may be concern about giving a prolonged course of unpleasant and potentially dangerous treatment. The temptation is to give smaller doses, switch quickly to oral preparations, avoid more toxic agents and to shorten the course of treatment. Such compassion is misconceived. Multiple pathology and atypical symptoms make it difficult to follow the clinical progress of the disease. Again, impaired immunological function increases the importance of achieving complete bacterial irradication. Antibacterial therapy thus has to be particularly vigorous in an elderly patient. If he has severe mental and physical incapacity it may be best not to embark on it.

Since many old people have heart valve defects, and many are in need of dental surgery and genito-urinary or gastro-intestinal instrumentation there are frequent instances in which prophylactic antibiotic treatment might be considered. A combination of 1 mega-unit of benzylpenicillin and 0.6 mega-units of procaine penicillin should be given 30 min before a dental procedure. Again, cystoscopy, sigmoidoscopy, or colonoscopy perhaps should be preceded by 2 mega-units of benzylpenicillin and 80 mg gentamycin. Unfortunately, there is little hard information on the incidence of endocarditis in elderly patients when this is not done. Clinicians thus are likely to use antibiotics where there is breathlessness associated with mitral stenosis or a previous history of valve replacement surgery. They are less likely to embark on this in someone with an asymptomatic aortic sclerosis, or mild mitral incompetence.

References

Anturane Reinfarction Trial Research Group (1980) Sulphinpyrazone in the prevention of sudden death after myocardial infarction. New Engl J Med 302: 250–256

Burr ML, King S, Davies HEF, Pathy MS (1977) The effects of discontinuing long-term diuretic therapy in the elderly. Age Ageing 6: 38–45

Currie G, MacNeill RM, Walker JG, Barrie E, Mudie EW (1974) Medical and social screening of patients aged 70 to 72 by an urban general practice health team. Br Med J 2: 108–111

Dall JLC (1981) Observations on the action of digoxin. In: Caird FI, Grimley Evans J (eds) Advanced Geriatric medicine, Pitman, London, pp 56–61

Greenblatt DJ, Duhme DW, Allen MD, Koch-Weser J (1977) Clinical toxicity of frusemide in hospitalised patients. A report from the Boston Collaborative Drug Surveillance Program. Am Heart J 94: 6–13

Hjalmarson A, Herlitz J, Malek I, Ryden L, Vedin A, Waldenstrom A, Wedel H, Elmfeldt D, Holmberg S, Nyberg G, Swedberg K, Waagstern F, Waldenstrom J, Wilhelmson L, Wilhelmson C (1981) Effect on mortality of metoprolol in acute myocardial infarction. Lancet 2: 823–826

Johnston GD, Kelly JG, McDevitt DG (1978) Do patients take digoxin? Br Med J 40: 1–7

Law R, Chalmers C (1976) Medicines and elderly people: a general practice survey. Br Med J 1: 565–568

MacDonald A (1979) The management of infective endocarditis. Br J Hosp Med 21: 498–510
McHaffie D, Purcell H, Mitchell-Heggs P, Guy A (1978) QJM 47: 401–402
Norwegian Multicentre Study Group (1981) Timolol-induced reduction in mortality and infarction.
    New Engl J Med 304: 801–807

4 Disorders of the Vascular System

Hypertension

Rationale for Treatment

The mean systolic and diastolic blood pressures of elderly men and women are substantially higher than those recorded in young adults (Fig. 4.1). Over the age of 65, however, there is no further increase with age. Indeed, in patients who are sick and disabled there actually is a decline of blood pressure in extreme old age. The question arises as to whether hypertension is an inevitable concomitant of ageing. There are people in whom blood pressures do not increase with age.

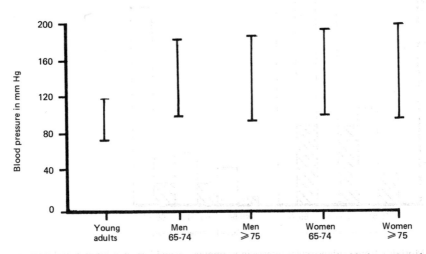

Fig. 4.1. Mean systolic and diastolic pressures of young adults and elderly men and women (MacLennan et al. 1980).

Examples include some Pacific and African populations living in separation from Western society.

Where the blood pressure is elevated in old age, there is debate as to whether this is harmful. In Framingham, USA, the risk of hypertension causing death from cardiovascular disease increases with the age of the subjects in both men and women (Fig. 4.2). Contrary to widespread belief, the systolic pressure is at least as important as the diastolic one as a risk factor in the elderly. There is a similar association between hypertension and morbidity, so that elderly patients with hypertension are more likely to suffer from coronary artery disease, intermittent claudication, atherothrombotic brain infarction, and congestive heart failure.

Even if hypertension causes harm to old people, the question remains as to whether treatment will reverse the adverse effects of the condition. In one investigation, effective control of hypertension halved morbidity in men aged 60 years and over. The total numbers were small, however, so that there is doubt as to the validity of the conclusions. The study most likely to provide an answer is that conducted by a European Working Party on High Blood Pressure in the Elderly. Here a large number of elderly patients on treatment for hypertension are being compared with a control group of hypertensives on no treatment.

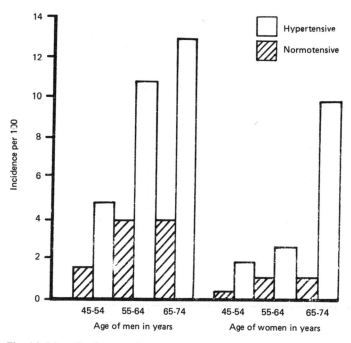

Fig. 4.2. Mortality from cardiovascular disease in normotensive and hypertensive men and women (Kannel 1976).

Though the study has now been running for several years, no differences in mortality or morbidity have been reported yet.

The potential benefits of hypotensive therapy have to be balanced against its very real dangers. Reduced distensibility in the aorta and large arteries of old people causes a widening gap between systolic and diastolic pressures. In this situation a relatively minor fall in the diastolic pressure may produce a catastrophic drop in the systolic one. A further problem is that baroreceptor reflexes are impaired in old age, so that hypotensive drugs are more likely to produce wild swings in the blood pressure and to cause postural hypotension. Added to this is the fact that hypertension interferes with the ability of cerebral circulation to vasodilate in response to changes in perfusion. This means that hypotension is more likely to give rise to dizziness, light-headedness, falls, or even transient ischaemic attacks and cerebral infarction in the elderly.

At present there can be no firm guidelines on the treatment of hypertension in the elderly, so that current policies are based on clinical experience and prejudice. The question arises as to what a doctor hopes to achieve by controlling hypertension. In symptomless hypertension in a man of 80 there is little point in trying to bring about a marginal increase in his life expectancy. If, on the other hand, a reduction in blood pressure prevented him from becoming chairfast as the result of a stroke, it would be a great practical benefit. The balance, therefore, would seem to be in favour of treating hypertension even in extreme old age.

Consideration should also be given to the level of blood pressure which should be treated. Certainly, patients with a diastolic pressure in excess of 105 mm Hg are much more likely to benefit than those with more modest hypertension (Veterans Administration Comparative Study Group on Anti-hypertensive Agents 1972). Age, on the other hand, increases rather than diminishes the importance of hypertension as a risk, and systolic pressures assume increasing relevance. If hypertension were to be treated at all in the elderly, then a systolic pressure of 160 mm Hg and a diastolic one of 90 mm Hg might be more appropriate starting points.

The physical condition of the patient also has a bearing on whether to treat hypertension. Though it seems rational to identify and treat the condition before it has had time to cause target organ damage, many patients present for the first time with a stroke, left ventricular failure, or chronic renal failure. Injudicious treatment of such people with hypotensive drugs may exacerbate rather than control symptoms. Even if there is no aggravation, treatment may not be of much benefit. An example is that in one trial of hypotensive therapy in stroke patients of 65 and over, a reduction of the diastolic pressure had only a marginal effect, and control of the systolic pressure had no effect on morbidity or mortality (Carter 1970). Where there is evidence of severe target organ damage therefore it seems reasonable to limit treatment to patients with diastolic pressure in excess of 110 mm Hg and to ignore the systolic pressure. A caveat is that such recommendations may well be changed in the light of increasing information on hypertension in old age.

The general prognosis for the patient also is important. There may be no point in trying to prolong the life of a patient with severe multi-infarct dementia. An old woman with carcinoma of the breast, however, may have a life expectancy only marginally less than that of a healthy counterpart. Here, control of incidental hypertension may prevent the disability of a cerebrovascular accident.

General Principles of Management

In deciding to treat hypertension the first essential is to establish that it really is present. Old people, as a result of changes in the regulatory system, have blood pressures which are even more labile than those of young adults. It is important to take a series of recumbent pressure readings under conditions of minimal stress before deciding that hypertension requires attention. Treatment then should commence by using the smallest recommended dose of a particular drug. Both lying and standing pressures should then be monitored to ensure that the patient does not develop postural hypotension.

Certain hypotensive agents should not be used in the elderly. Adrenergic neurone blocking agents, including bethanidine, debrisoquine, and guanethidine, paralyse the normal responses to an erect posture. This is particularly dangerous in old age, where autonomic reflexes may be seriously compromised already. If these drugs are used in old age a high incidence of falls, strokes, and broken proximal femurs can be guaranteed.

Clonidine has the advantage over adrenergic blocking agents that it does not cause postural hypotension. Undesirable effects include sedation, fatigue, headache, and a dry mouth. In old people disturbances in sleep, vivid nightmares, and even agitated depression can be particularly troublesome. Quite apart from these, there is the danger that sudden withdrawal may cause a serious rebound hypertension. In patients where compliance is a problem this is a major disadvantage.

Methyldopa also acts centrally by interfering with the sympathetic drive. Unlike clonidine, it can cause postural hypotension and often does so in the elderly. Neurological complications include sedation, drowsiness, fatigue, and forgetfulness. Particularly troublesome in old people is a 5%–10% incidence of depression. Again, it very occasionally may precipitate Parkinsonism, though more usually it simply has been given coincidentally to a patient developing the disorder. Despite these problems the drug has been used widely and successfully in old age. In recent years, however, it has increasingly been replaced by beta-adrenergic blocking agents.

The long-term treatment of hypertension poses certain practical problems. Non-compliance is a common reason for a poor response. Again, before deciding that a drug is ineffective it should be pushed to the maximum possible dosage. Doctors often resort to other drugs before an attempt has been made to achieve a maximal response from the initial one. This approach leads to polypharmacy, with further problems of compliance. When these two issues are tackled, many cases of apparent resistance to hypotensive agents disappear.

Diuretics

Thiazide diuretics are used widely as the drugs of first choice in the treatment of hypertension. As such they are capable of achieving adequate control in up to 70% of patients with mild to moderate hypertension. They achieve this by reducing the amount of sodium, chloride, and water within the intravascular compartment.

The side-effects of thiazide diuretics are discussed in Chap. 3, but some of these require particular emphasis in relation to their use as hypotensive agents. One of these is that they cause hypokalaemia. This can be treated by giving potassium supplements, but much of the mineral given in this way is excreted immediately by the kidneys, so that daily doses of up to 60 mmol may be required to correct blood levels. An alternative and less cumbersome approach is to give a potassium-sparing agent along with the thiazide. Such drugs enhance the diuretic effect of the latter while balancing its kaluretic one. Diuretics may cause postural hypotension by the over-vigorous elimination of sodium and chloride. Since the mechanisms reducing the blood pressure and causing postural hypotension are the same, the only remedy is to reduce the dose of thiazide. In some instances an additional cause of the postural hypotension may be potassium depletion, requiring treatment with supplements or potassium-sparing agents.

A final practical difficulty is that a diuretic may cause urinary incontinence. This is likely to happen in a patient with a prolapse, prostatism, or a neurogenic bladder, or whose mobility is restricted by locomotor or neurological disease. In this situation beta-blocking agents may become the hypotensive agents of first choice.

Beta-adrenoceptor Blocking Agents

All beta-blocking agents have a hypotensive effect. Several mechanisms may be involved. One suggestion was that hypotension is the result of a reduced pulse rate and stroke volume. In patients treated with beta-blockers, however, there is no correlation between the fall in pulse rate and the fall in blood pressure, suggesting that factors other than a reduced cardiac output are important. The effect of beta-blockers on plasma renin concentrations also has been investigated, but reports vary on the relationship, if any, between initial plasma renin levels and the hypotensive response to beta-blockers. Finally, the hypotensive effect of beta-blockers might be mediated through suppression of sympathetic activity in the hypothalamus and midbrain. This may be fortunate for old people since, despite their low cardiac output and reduced plasma renin concentrations, they usually show a brisk hypotensive response to beta-blockers.

All beta-blockers produce side-effects, but these are more prominent with some than with others. Their effect on cardiac output can be catastrophic in patients with congestive cardiac failure. Since a quarter of people over the age of 65 years have ischaemic heart disease it is wise to monitor all of those on beta-blockers for signs of fluid retention until dosage, pulse rate, and blood pressure have been stabilised. A low cardiac output reduces the blood supply to the hands and feet, inducing Raynaud's phenomenon in susceptible individuals. In elderly diabetics or heavy smokers it may precipitate frank gangrene. There also may be a dramatic fall in the pulse rate, but this can safely be ignored if the patient remains in sinus rhythm, and there are no symptoms such as faintness, dizziness, or falls. Beta-blockers hardly ever cause postural hypotension.

Since both hypertension and diabetes mellitus are common in old people, the possibility of an interaction with hypoglycaemic agents is particularly relevant to them. Beta-blockers reduce blood glucose levels by suppressing the catecholamine secretion. Usually, however, the effects are minor, so that beta-blockers rarely cause hypoglycaemic attacks in diabetics.

A more important problem is that beta-blockers may mask autonomic manifestations of hypoglycaemia, such as sweating and tachycardia. Age-related changes in the autonomic nervous system compound this, so that hypoglycaemia in an old person on propranolol may present as a vague drowsiness and memory impairment. Failure to recognise the serious import of the condition can lead to permanent cortical destruction.

Suppression of sympathetic activity in the central nervous system may have serious consequences. Patients of any age may be troubled by sleep disturbances and vivid dreams, but old people sometimes go into a state of confusion, disorientation, and agitation. This resolves rapidly when the beta-blocker is withdrawn. A numerically more common problem is that beta-blockers may cause depression. A large proportion of patients on propranolol develop depressive symptoms, and the incidence of these increases with the duration and dosage of therapy. In view of the high incidence of depression with age, it is important to keep the condition in mind when reviewing an elderly patient on a beta-blocker.

Susceptible individuals may develop bronchospasm in response to beta-adrenoceptor blockade, but this is no more of a problem in the elderly than in any other group. It would be interesting, indeed, to see whether age-related changes in immunological and respiratory function perhaps decreased rather than increased the bronchoconstrictor response to beta-blockers.

If a clinician decides to use a beta-blocker he then is faced with a formidable array of alternatives. The pharmaceutical explosion has been the result of a search for drugs which affect cardiac function without altering smooth muscle function or the tissue response to insulin. Hope that this might be possible is based on the observation that heart muscle contains high concentrations of beta-1 receptors, whereas smooth muscle and liver contain high levels of beta-2 receptors. Drugs with a high affinity for beta-1 receptors would be expected to produce cardiac effects with minimal bronchial or vascular side-effects.

No drugs have complete beta-1 selectivity, but a large number have partial selectivity (Table 4.1). The main role for selective agents is in the management of patients with a history of bronchospasm. They also have marginal advantages in diabetes mellitus. Their advantages as hypotensive agents are more marginal. Thus, though they are more likely to control hypertension during episodes of stress, they are no more effective than non-selective agents at lowering resting pressures. This pharmacological effect is unlikely to be of great

Table 4.1. Beta-adrenergic blocking agents which are non-selective, cardioselective, and have partial agonist activity (PAA)

Non-selective agents	Selective agents	Agents with PAA
Propranolol	Atenolol	Oxprenolol
Oxprenolol	Metoprolol	Pindolol
Sotalol	Acebutolol	Alprenolol
Alprenolol		Acebutolol
Timolol		
Nadolol		

importance to a chairbound old lady receiving a high level of care from her daughter.

Some agents which block beta-adrenergic receptors also have a mild stimulant effect on the same receptors. The theoretical advantage of this is that though these drugs are equally effective in controlling hypertension, they are less likely than other beta-blockers to precipitate cardiac failure. They have no advantages over other agents in the elderly. They might be used in a patient with cardiac failure, but though causing less myocardial depression, they do still cause this to some extent and should be used with extreme caution.

The effects of ageing on renal and hepatic function modify the dosage of a beta-blocking agent required to achieve an effective blood level. A large proportion of lipid-soluble agents is metabolised by the liver before reaching the systemic circulation. This means that in old people where liver metabolism is impaired, much higher blood concentrations are achieved by much smaller oral doses. Examples of drugs affected in this way include propranolol, oxprenolol, metoprolol, and alprenolol.

Water-soluble agents are excreted unchanged in the kidneys. Dependent on the degree of renal impairment in an elderly patient, dosage of these drugs may also have to be reduced to keep blood levels within the normal range. Drugs in this group include atenolol, acebutolol, sotalol, and nadolol.

Another important aspect of dosage in the elderly is the frequency with which an agent should be given. Obviously, compliance would be improved if a once daily dose was effective in controlling hypertension. Even metoprolol, a drug with a relatively short half-life (2.9 h) can, if given once daily, achieve a control of hypertension which is almost as good as that obtained by a three times daily regime. The only differences are that the more frequent dosage is slightly more potent and produces fewer fluctuations in level. Propranolol has similar efficacy in hypertension when given once daily. The evidence, then, is that even though the half-life of many beta-blocking agents is short, their therapeutic effects outlive this. Old people with hypertension could thus be treated with, say, 80–160 mg propranolol or oxprenolol once daily.

Another approach would be to use drugs with a prolonged duration of action. Examples include acebutolol, atenolol, nadolol, and sotalol. Information on their use in the elderly is relatively limited, and it would seem important for investigators to establish firmly that cumulation is not a problem in old age. As yet, there is no positive evidence that this occurs.

It is also possible to prolong high levels of beta-blockers by formulating them in sustained release preparations. Both slow-release propranolol and slow-release oxprenolol are currently available. Further work is required to determine whether, in the elderly, beta-blockers with long half-lives or those in slow-release matrices have any major advantage over a single daily dose of short-half-life beta-blockers.

Opinions vary on the exact role and use of beta-blocking agents in the treatment of hypertension in the elderly. A reasonable approach is to use a beta-blocker along with a diuretic where the diuretic on its own has failed to control the hypertension. A situation in which it would be the drug of first choice would be where a patient suffered from urinary frequency or urgency. In most cases either propranolol or oxprenolol would be acceptable as the beta-blocker. Selective beta-blockers would be required only if there was chronic obstructive airways disease, and there should rarely be a need for agents with intrinsic sympatheticomimetic activity, particularly if beta-blockers are normally given with a diuretic. Finally, there is very little evidence that beta-blockers with a long half-life or in slow-release matrices have much advantage over those with a short half-life, even where these are given only once daily.

Vasodilators

If the combination of a thiazide diuretic and a beta-blocking agent does not control hypertension, the use of a peripheral vasodilator should be considered. Such a drug is of limited use if given alone. This is because the hypotension caused by dilatation stimulates an increased sympathetic drive which returns the blood pressure almost to pre-treatment levels. In old people with a poor coronary circulation, an increased sympathetic drive may produce unpleasant symptoms such as palpitations and chest pain. Beta-blockers prevent this happening by paralysing the reflex. Thus, they both potentiate the hypotensive effect of the vasodilator and eliminate its side-effects. Another advantage of combined therapy is that it rarely causes postural hypotension, presumably because the peripheral arteriolar response to adrenaline or noradrenaline is unaffected. The vasodilator most widely used in the treatment of hypertension is hydralazine. Apart from its effects on the cardiovascular system, the adverse effect giving rise to most concern is its propensity to cause systemic lupus erythematosis. Around one-half of patients on long-term treatment with hydralazine in excess of 200 mg/day develop positive anti-nuclear factor in their peripheral blood. With doses of less than 200 mg/day the incidence of anti-nuclear factor is only marginally greater than that in the general population. The dose in old people should start at 25 mg/day, increasing progressively up to a maximum of 150 mg/day.

Another vasodilator used in the treatment of hypertension is prazosin. It has the advantage over hydralazine that it does not cause a reflex tachycardia. Unfortunately, it may cause postural hypotension and fluid retention. Further clinical experience, therefore, is required before the drug can be recommended for use in the elderly.

The calcium antagonists verapamil and nifedipine have a vasodilator effect on the peripheral circulation, and are effective in reducing both systolic and diastolic pressures in hypertensive patients. Side-effects include flushing, palpitations, and dizziness, but these are minimised by giving the drugs along with beta-adrenergic blocking agents. If early trials suggesting efficacy and freedom from serious side-effects are confirmed, these drugs should have a useful role to play in the management of hypertension in the elderly.

Captopril promotes peripheral vasodilatation by inhibiting the enzyme responsible for the conversion of angiotensin I to angiotensin II. It has a potent hypotensive effect and has been used in the short-term and long-term control of hypertension. There is a high incidence of side-effects, which include skin rashes, taste disturbances, dizziness, vertigo, leucopenia, and nephrotic syndrome. This can be reduced by sticking to a maximum dose of 25 mg three times a day. However, further evidence of its safety is required before it can be recommended for routine use in old people.

Combination Therapy

Treatment of hypertension in old age requires a general strategy. A reasonable one is to commence with a thiazide diuretic. If, on its own, this is ineffective, a beta-blocking agent should be added. Where this approach works, medication can be simplified by using formulations of the two preparations in one tablet (Table 4.2). The initial dose of beta-blocker may be inadequate, in which case the dose of this alone should be increased. This means that combination formulations should only be used if the initial doses of diuretic and beta-blocker achieve adequate control. Where a combination of diuretic and beta-blocker is ineffective, a vasodilator should be added. At present, the most widely used one remains hydralazine.

Table 4.2 Formulations which combine thiazide diuretics with beta-blocking agents

Diuretic			Beta-blocker	
Metoprolol	100 mg	+	Hydrochlorothiazide	12.5 mg
Nadolol	40 mg	+	Bendrofluazide	5 mg
Propranolol	80 mg	+	Bendrofluazide	2.5 mg
Timolol	10 mg	+	Bendrofluazide	2.5 mg
Acebutolol	200 mg	+	Hydrochlorothiazide	12.5 mg
Sotalol	160 mg	+	Hydrochlorothiazide	25 mg
Oxprenolol	160 mg	+	Cyclopenthiazide	250 μg
Pindolol	10 mg	+	Clopamide	5 mg
Atenolol	50 mg	+	Chlorthalidone	12.5 mg

Postural Hypotension

A large proportion of even healthy old people experience a fall in systolic blood pressure when rising from a recumbent position to a standing position. This is partly related to degenerative changes found in the autonomic nervous system in old age. In addition, changes in the elasticity of blood vessels may interfere with both baroreceptor function and the response of blood vessels to autonomic stimulation. Postural hypotension is even more common in sick old people, in whom a wide range of other factors accentuate deficiencies in the autonomic nervous system and blood vessels (Table 4.3).

Table 4.3. Causes of postural hypotension in the elderly

Inadequate cardiac output

Myocardial ischaemia or valvular disease

Inadequate peripheral resistance

Drugs (ganglion blocking agents, phenothiazines,
    tricyclic antidepressants, anticholinergic agents,
    levodopa, and barbiturates)

Lesions of the peripheral nervous system

Diabetic autonomic neuropathy

Parkinson's disease

Lesions of the central nervous system

Cerebrovascular disease

Diminished blood volume

Haemorrhage

Dehydration

Diuretic therapy

Prolonged immobility

The treatment of postural hypotension is dependent on its causes. Thus, patients with myocardial ischaemia or valvular disease may respond to cardiac glycosides. Discontinuation of drugs affecting the autonomic nervous system also often produces a dramatic recovery. Where diabetes mellitus is kept under careful control, changes in the autonomic nervous system are less likely to be progressive. Unfortunately, most drugs used in treating Parkinson's disease accentuate rather than relieve postural hypotension. Correction of blood loss or fluid and electrolyte loss also should alleviate postural hypotension. Finally, gentle but firm gradual mobilisation of a convalescent elderly patient is necessary to recondition his orthostatic reflexes.

Once these measures have been taken there remains a group of patients who persist in having postural hypotension. Many old people have wide fluctuations in blood pressure without experiencing any symptoms. Those who do have attacks of dizziness, black-outs, or falls usually have intracerebral disease in which there is a breakdown of autoregulation in cerebral blood flow. The most common cause of this is cerebrovascular degeneration.

Even if patients have symptoms it is important to perform measurements under standard conditions. The patient should be standing for at least 2 min before a pressure is taken, and the drop in systolic pressure should be at least 20 mm Hg. After this, pressures should be recorded for at least a week before deciding that the disorder is persistent and requires treatment.

The wide range of compounds which have been tried in postural hypotension is a reflection that treatment of the condition often is unsatisfactory. The drug most widely used is the mineralocorticoid fludrocortisone. In small doses it increases the sensitivity of effector sites to noradrenaline and thus causes peripheral vasoconstriction. Though this is its main mode of action it inevitably also causes fluid retention. Since a large proportion of old people have overt or latent heart disease, fludrocortisone often produces peripheral oedema or more serious signs of congestive cardiac failure. The drug also causes potassium depletion and potassium supplements should always be given along with it. Dosage should start at 0.1 mg daily, increasing this by 0.1 mg every 5 days until the blood pressure and, more important, the symptoms are controlled. The maximum dose is 1.0 mg daily, but many old people do not reach this before they exhibit signs of serious fluid retention.

A more hazardous approach is to give a monoamine oxidase inhibitor along with tyramine-containing foods. The unpredictability of the blood pressure response and the disasters possible if the blood pressure rises too high, limit its usefulness.

An alternative is to block the synthesis of prostaglandins, agents with a peripheral vasodilator effect. Indomethacin, in doses of 75–150 mg/day, sometimes is effective here, but is likely to be associated with severe side-effects.

Drugs designed to mimic the effect of noradrenaline might be expected to benefit patients with postural hypotension. Unfortunately, sympatheticomimetic drugs are of no value in this condition and often produce intolerable side-effects, which include tremor, tachycardia, and sweating. Another way of producing peripheral vasoconstriction would be to use a beta-blocking agent. Any benefit, however, would be balanced by the effect which the drug had on reducing the cardiac output. A solution to the problem might be to use a beta-blocker with intrinsic sympatheticomimetic activity. Though such a drug, pindolol, was used with success in three patients with severe orthostatic hypotension, further experience is required before this can be recommended as a useful approach to postural hypotension in the elderly.

While drugs may be useful in controlling postural hypotension, it is important also to advise on physical measures. These include sleeping with the bed tilted head upwards, performing regular postural exercises, and applying graduated pressure to the lower limbs with specially designed tights or even a pressure suit.

Peripheral Vascular Disease

A large number of old people have arterial occlusive disease presenting as absent pedal pulses and cold, often cyanosed feet. Only a minority suffer from symptoms such as intermittent claudication or rest pain, and an even smaller group go on to develop frank necrosis and gangrene. Reconstructive arterial surgery rarely is useful in old people since most of them have multiple areas of occlusion, affecting small as well as large vessels.

There is the temptation to show evidence of concern and therapeutic activity by prescribing a peripheral arterial dilator. This, however, is of little value in peripheral arteriosclerosis because affected arteries are rigid and thus unresponsive to neuronal or chemical stimulation. Indeed, vasodilators may open up unaffected vessels, and thus divert blood away from the ischaemic area supplied by a sclerotic one. As a counter to this argument, manufacturers have provided evidence that some vasodilators improve blood flow by coincidentally reducing blood viscosity and resistance to flow through small vessels. Some of them are still widely used, but controlled trials have failed to establish their benefit over placebo when given for either rest pain or intermittent claudication.

Vasodilators also have been used to heal overt or impending necrosis. There are many anecdotes of a dramatic response to an intravenous or even an intra-arterial infusion of such drugs. Convincing evidence on efficacy, however, has not been documented yet. Table 4.4 lists some of the drugs in current use for peripheral vascular disease.

Many old people with peripheral vascular disease do not suffer from intermittent claudication, simply because they are not sufficiently mobile. This does not prevent them from suffering from intractable rest pain. Since ischaemic pain is related partly to the release of prostaglandins, there is a theoretical basis for using a prostaglandin inhibitor. There is limited evidence that agents such as ibuprofen are effective in relieving rest pain, but further experience of this approach is required.

If the pain results from frank necrosis, the only treatment is amputation. Sometimes, however, the patient refuses surgery, or is so ill that surgery would inevitably be fatal. In this situation adequate doses of a narcotic analgesic should be given. The rules should be the same as in terminal cancer, namely that the dose should be large enough to relieve pain and given on a regular basis frequently enough to prevent the recurrence of pain (Chap. 12).

Table 4.4. Drugs used for the treatment of peripheral vascular disease

Drug	Mode of action	Route of administration
Nicotinic acid derivatives	Vasodilators	Oral
Inositol	Vasodilator	Oral
Oxpentifylline	Vasodilator (alpha-antagonist) Reduced blood viscosity	Oral
Naftidrofuryl	Vasodilator Increased glucose uptake	Oral Intravenous Intra-arterial
Cyclandelate	Vasodilator	Oral
Tolazoline	Vasodilator (alpha-blocker)	Oral
Thymoxamine	Vasodilator (alpha-blocker)	Oral
Phenoxybenzamine	Vasodilator (alpha-blocker)	Oral
Isoxuprine	Vasodilator (beta-agonist)	Oral Intramuscular Intravenous Intra-arterial

Deep Leg Vein Thrombosis and Pulmonary Embolism

Prophylaxis

In the population at large, age has only a marginal effect on the incidence of deep leg vein thrombosis (Fig. 4.3). Many old people, however, suffer from conditions in which deep leg vein thrombosis is particularly prevalent. Examples are that around 40% of patients with a fractured neck of femur have venographic evidence of a thrombosis, and that up to 50% of patients with a hemiparesis have positive radioactive fibrinogen scans in the lower limb affected by the stroke. Other factors which increase the risk of thrombosis in old age are disorders causing prolonged pooling of blood in the legs, such as congestive cardiac failure, varicose veins, or immobility due to locomotor or neurological conditions. Illnesses increasing the coagulability of the blood include carcinomatosis, dehydration, and acute or chronic inflammation. The last-mentioned embraces such diverse disorders as bronchopneumonia, urinary tract infections, cellulitis, and myocardial infarction.

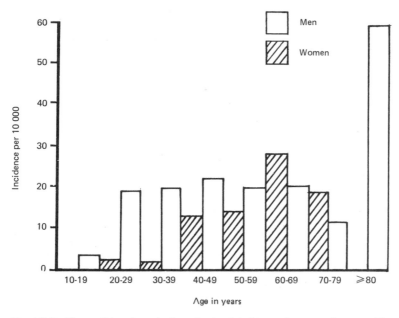

Fig. 4.3. Incidence of deep leg vein thrombosis related to age in men and women (Coon et al. 1973).

If patients are at increased risk, the question arises as to whether the risk should be reduced by using anticoagulants. Unfortunately the treatment of such a large and heterogeneous group of elderly patients with prophylactic anti-coagulants would create insurmountable dangers and difficulties. Fortunately, perhaps, there is no evidence that anticoagulants reduce mortality in patients over 65 with myocardial infarctions or in patients with strokes of any age. Again patients with dehydration or acute infections are best managed by treating the primary disorder. There is the possibility that old people with congestive cardiac failure would benefit from anticoagulants, but there is no clinical evidence to confirm or refute this. This leaves patients with a fractured proximal femur or about to undergo other major forms of surgery. In one study of patients over 40 having major operations, only one out of 2045 patients on anticoagulant therapy died from thrombo-embolic disease. In 2076 patients not on an anticoagulant 16 died from this. Although 158 of those on an anticoagulant compared with 117 of the controls developed a wound haematoma, there was no difference in the haemoglobin levels, blood transfusion requirements, or death rates from haemorrhage in the two groups.

If it is decided to use anticoagulant prophylaxis in old people with a fractured proximal femur or undergoing major surgery, the agent of choice is heparin. This is given subcutaneously in a dose of 5000 units 2 h before operation, and thereafter eight-hourly for 7 days.

Oral anticoagulants could also be used in this situation, but they are less effective than subcutaneous heparin. The need to make regular checks on prothrombin times also makes them more difficult to use. The sugar, dextran 70 also is effective in prophylaxis against thrombosis. It is given at the time of surgery as a 4-h infusion of 500 ml dextran 70. This is repeated on the first and second postoperative days. It is debatable whether intravenous dextran 70 or subcutaneous heparin is easier to administer. The major advantage of heparin over dextran is that it gives a lower incidence of deep leg vein thrombosis.

Treatment of Deep Leg Vein Thrombosis

The first problem in treating deep leg vein thrombosis is making the correct diagnosis. One-third of patients with clinical signs of the disorder have normal veins. Again many patients with thrombosis, particularly of the pelvic and femoral veins, may not exhibit clinical evidence of it. A counsel of perfection would be to perform phlebography on all patients at risk from or suspected of having the condition. The technique, however, is specialised and time-consuming and as such unlikely to be used routinely on all potential candidates passing through a geriatric unit. Radioactive fibrinogen scans are easier to perform, but there is considerable doubt as to the clinical relevance of a positive test. Finally, ultrasonography is simple, but totally inaccurate. Most clinicians, then, will continue to treat deep vein thrombosis on the basis of clinical findings.

The next decision is which drug to use. If the patient has had a cerebral haemorrhage and is thus at risk of having a further bleed from heparin and an oral anticoagulant, then phenylbutazone, which by virtue of its effect on prostaglandin synthesis has a mild anticoagulant effect, may be used in this situation. Phenylbutazone itself is very toxic, however, so that the risks of death from pulmonary embolism have to be balanced against the risks of fluid retention or gastro-intestinal haemorrhage. A safer policy is simply to treat the pain associated with the thrombosis using a less toxic analgesic, such as ibuprofen or naproxen.

Anticoagulants should never be withheld on the basis of age alone. The drug which most rapidly reduces the coagulability of blood is heparin. This is best given as an initial 5000-unit bolus and then a continuous intravenous infusion in a dose of 10 000 units 12-hourly in 500 ml of 5% dextrose. Heparin usually is given coincidentally with an oral anticoagulant and continued until the latter has brought the prothrombin time to the desired level. The clotting time should be checked at the start of treatment, and rechecked daily thereafter. The ideal for this is twice the control value.

The indanedione and coumarin oral anticoagulants reduce blood coagulation by interfering with the hepatic synthesis of prothrombin, factor VII, factor IX, and factor X. Ageing has a pronounced effect on the sensitivity of patients to oral anticoagulants. Thus much lower doses of warfarin should be given to old people to produce changes in prothrombin activity equivalent to those in the young. There is no change in the metabolism or protein binding of warfarin with age, and the alteration results from a change in the sensitivity to warfarin of clotting factor synthesis. The practical implication is that much smaller loading and maintenance doses of anticoagulants should be used in elderly patients. On average, doses should be 30%–40% lower than in younger patients. This would give a loading dose for warfarin of 20 mg followed by a maintenance dose of between 2 and 6 mg daily. Treatment, once started, should be continued for 3–6 months.

The situation is even more complex if the elderly patient is suffering from disorders known to impair elimination, change protein binding, or increase hepatic sensitivity to anticoagulants. These include subnutrition, acute illness, pyrexia, hepatobiliary disease, renal impairment, congestive cardiac failure, and thyrotoxicosis. Another factor complicating anticoagulant control is concurrent drug treatment. Table 4.5 lists some of the drugs more commonly used in the elderly which interfere with oral anticoagulant activity. Agents including phenytoin, phenobarbitone, carbamazepine, and alcohol actually reduce anticoagulant efficacy by induction of the hepatic enzymes responsible for anticoagulant metabolism. Finally, anticoagulants may increase the activity of other drugs by interfering with their metabolism. Examples are that they enhance the hypoglycaemic effects of tolbutamide and chlorpropamide and increase the sedative effect of phenytoin.

Anticoagulant control also poses many practical problems in mentally or physically frail elderly patients. There are the obvious ones of poor compliance or failure to follow advice on concurrent medication. Again, regular attendance at an anticoagulant clinic may be difficult to arrange, particularly at times when the ambulance or hospital car service is disrupted by weather or industrial action. These considerations mean that there are times when anticoagulant therapy should be withdrawn gradually before discharge from hospital, rather than after the theoretically ideal interval.

Table 4.5. Drugs increasing oral anticoagulant activity

Drug	Mode of action
Broad-spectrum antibiotics (e.g. ampicillin, tetracycline)	Reduction in bacterial synthesis of vitamin K
Chloral derivatives	Displacement from albumin
Phenylbutazone	Displacement from albumin Inhibition of coagulation
Salicylates	Inhibitors of coagulation
Thyroxine	Increased degradation of clotting factors
Sulphonamides	Displacement from albumin

Treatment of Pulmonary Embolism

In the elderly, pulmonary embolism often is left untreated because it is not diagnosed. Though it can present with chest pain and haemoptysis, it often presents with less specific symptoms such as confusion, drowsiness, loss of mobility, weakness, dizziness, or mild breathlessness. A high index of suspicion is required therefore.

Treatment with anticoagulants is essentially that for deep leg vein thrombosis. In addition it might be necessary to give oxygen, treat shock, and control pain. Where the embolism is massive and has blocked a major vein, surgery and thrombolytic therapy may be necessary. Whether or not these are used depends upon the quality of the patient's life before the embolism, upon the long-term prognosis, and upon the prospects of him surviving with his mental function intact.

References

Carter J (1970) A trial of long-term hypotensive therapy in cerebrovascular disease. Lancet 1: 485–489

Coon WW, Willis PW, Keller JB (1973) Venous thrombo-embolism and other venous diseases in the Tecumseh Community Health Study. Circulation 48: 839–846

International Multicentre Trial (1975) Prevention of fatal postoperative pulmonary embolism by low doses of heparin. Lancet 2: 45–51

Kannel WB (1976) Blood pressure and the development of cardiovascular disease in the aged. In: Caird FI, Dall JLC, Kennedy RD (eds) Cardiology in old age, Plenum, New York

MacLennan WJ, Hall MRP, Timothy JI (1980) Postural hypotension in old age: is it a disorder of the nervous system or of blood vessels? Age Ageing 9: 25–32

Veterans Administration Comparative Study Group on Anti-hypertensive Agents (1972) Effects of treatment on morbidity in hypertension III. Influence of age, diastolic pressure and prior cardiovascular disease; further analysis of side effects. Circulation 45: 999–1004

5 Respiratory Disease

Pulmonary Function

A decline in connective tissue elasticity and increase in chest wall rigidity results in a decline in pulmonary function in the elderly which includes an increase in residual volume, decrease in pulmonary compliance, and an increase in closing volume. These changes in closing volume and compliance lead, in turn, to a decrease in arterial oxygen tension. The result is that a 60-year-old man would have to increase energy expenditure by 20% to achieve the same expansion against elastic recoil as a 20-year-old person. This leads in turn to an age-related decline in respiratory reserve.

There have been studies into the pulmonary function of healthy adults which relate pulmonary function to age (Table 5.1). Tidal volume, frequency of breathing and functional residual capacity remain unchanged, but residual volume increases markedly in old age, as do the lung clearance index and mixing

Table 5.1. $FEV_{1.0}$, FVC, and $FEV_{1.0}\%$ in older men and women (Milne and Williamson 1972)

	$FEV_{1.0}$ (l)		FVC (l)		$FEV_{1.0}\%$	
	Mean	SD	Mean	SD	Mean	SD
Men						
62–69	2.2	0.8	3.2	0.9	69	14
70–79	1.9	0.7	2.8	0.8	67	17
80+	2.0	0.5	2.9	0.7	69	11
Women						
62–69	1.6	0.5	2.0	0.6	81	10
70–79	1.4	0.5	1.8	0.5	81	13
80+	1.0	0.4	1.4	0.4	74	17

ratio. Cardio-respiratory fitness (maximum oxygen intake compared with body weight) shows a 20% decline between the ages of 50 and 70 years.

Though many elderly patients have emphysema it is wrong to use this as a marker of ageing. Cigarette smoking, air pollution, and underlying pulmonary disease—and not ageing—are the causes of emphysema in old age.

The prevalence of respiratory disease is high in old age. In a review of old people in the community in Glasgow, Caird and Akhtar (1972) found that 26% of men and 13% of women had chronic bronchitis, and that 9% of men and 4% of women had radiological evidence of tuberculosis.

Influenza

Influenza epidemics occur cyclically, usually in the autumn and winter. They can be caused by a well recognised virus strain, or by a new variant with different antigenic properties. The disorder can be devastating to the elderly population, where there is a high risk of serious complications and even death from the influenza infection. Since housebound old people rarely come in contact with outsiders, their risk of contracting influenza is low. Those in residential care, nursing homes, and hospitals run a much greater risk.

Immunisation against influenza infections has been shown to be effective in decreasing the development of influenza and pneumonia in the susceptible population, conferring immunity on up to 90% of the individuals vaccinated against that specific strain (Barker and Mulhooly 1980). Unfortunately, antigen drift occurs in influenza strains leading to new outbreaks, so that previous infections or immunisations do not confer effective immunity even to the same subtype if antigen variation is great enough. It is therefore essential that as an epidemic emerges the subtype is identified and appropriate immunisation against that subtype is undertaken in elderly persons to reduce the mortality and morbidity.

Influenza vaccination commonly produces mild side-effects. These include slight fever and malaise and local redness of the injection site. Serious side-effects are rare. There have been several reports of Guillain-Barré syndrome developing in some recipients of specific types of influenza vaccination. However, the risk of this after standard influenza vaccination is negligible and is not as great as that which would accompany illness from the influenza infection itself. Therefore, vaccination should be used to immunise the high-risk elderly person in the event of an influenza epidemic, provided that sufficient vaccine is available for the prevalent influenza subtype. There is no benefit in vaccinating with a previously prevalent subtype against the development of new subtypes.

There is, of course, the ethical dilemma of whether the vaccine should be given to patients with advanced physical or mental incapacity. The paramount consideration should be the quality of life as determined by the doctor, the relatives, and the patient himself.

Pneumonia

Diagnostic Considerations

Pneumonia is the commonest single terminal event in elderly patients. Its high prevalence is a result of a combination of factors, which include a diminished immune response and an inability to clear secretions from the chest. The latter may be the result of a cerebrovascular accident, over-enthusiastic sedation, or abdominal surgery. The presentation often is insidious, with apparently unrelated symptoms, such as acute confusion, reduced mobility, and drowsiness, without any pointer to the underlying pneumonia.

Clues to the organism causing the pneumonia may be present. For example, the patient may be known to be a chronic alcoholic or diabetic. As such he has an increased risk of infection with *Klebsiella pneumoniae*. Patients with long-standing chronic obstructive airways disease have an increased risk of *Haemophilus influenzae* infection. A recent viral infection, particularly influenza, frequently increases the risk of pneumonia due to *Streptococcus pyogenes*, whilst those patients who are immunosuppressed as part of the treatment of other conditions are often infected by opportunistic infections, including fungi.

The elderly patient who contracts pneumonia whilst in hospital tends to be infected with an organism that is currently prevalent in that environment. Often it is resistant to the commonly prescribed antibiotics. Where possible, culture and measurement of antibiotic sensitivity should be undertaken prior to commencement of therapy.

Management

Hydration

Dehydration is common usually as a result of poor fluid intake and increased loss resulting from fever or hyperventilation. There also is the problem that old people have a diminished renal reserve, so that even a minor fluid imbalance may be sufficient to precipitate severe uraemia. Great care must be taken therefore to ensure that the elderly patient is suitably hydrated, either orally or, if he is seriously ill, parenterally. Subcutaneous infusion often is adequate and less likely to cause fluid overload.

Treatment of Hypoxia

Hypoxia is a common respiratory complication of pneumonia accentuated both by a reduced pulmonary reserve and the increased incidence of chronic bronchitis and emphysema in old age. Caution should be exercised therefore not to promote hypoventilation associated with carbon dioxide retention in patients with severe underlying respiratory disease. This may be achieved by using a maximum 28% oxygen inhaled through an appropriate mask. Even at this concentration hypercapnia may occur, so that serial blood gas analyses may be required.

Treatment of Pain

Pleuritic pain is less common in older patients with pneumonia, but can occur. It should be treated with analgesia, but old people are sensitive to the central effects of narcotic agents. It often is difficult to achieve a balance between pain relief and serious respiratory depression.

Antibiotic Therapy

Choice of Drugs.   The choice for antibiotic therapy relies upon a "best guess" as to the suspected infecting organism. Sputum and blood samples should be sent off for culture, but while awaiting the results of these, a suitable broad-spectrum antibiotic should be given.

Broad-spectrum penicillins (amoxycillin or ampicillin) are useful as first-line drugs in pneumonia or exacerbations of chronic bronchitis. If *Staphylococcus aureus* is suspected, flucloxacillin should be added. Should the patient have penicillin sensitivity or fail to respond to amoxycillin or penicillin, then co-trimoxazole should be given. The cephalosporins are suitable and effective alternatives, but should be reserved for patients failing to respond to penicillins or co-trimoxazole. Most tetracyclines carry a risk of nephrotoxicity and should not be used in old people, most of whom have some degree of renal impairment. This also is a problem with many cephalosporins, but second-generation agents such as cefuroxime are free from this effect. Unfortunately, cefuroxime has to be given by injection.

Side-effects.   Apart from the well-documented hypersensitivity reactions, drugs of the penicillin group rarely have serious side-effects, but care must be exercised if they are prescribed in massive doses for elderly patients with poor renal function. Cumulation can occur, increasing the risk of toxicity from encephalopathy associated with cerebral irritation. Since most injectable penicillins contain either sodium or potassium salts, high doses may precipitate heart failure in patients with renal impairment.

Co-trimoxazole is used widely in the treatment of both chronic bronchitis and pneumonia, particularly in the elderly. Since the agent acts primarily by folic acid antagonism and since frail elderly patients are often mildly or frankly folic deficient, they are at particular risk of developing a full-blown deficiency picture with anaemia, neuropathy, and mental impairment. Rashes also are common and occasionally progress to the Stevens-Johnson syndrome (erythema multiforme) with renal failure and granulocyte depression. Other blood dyscrasias may occur but are less common. These well-documented side-effects make co-trimoxazole a drug of second choice in the treatment of pneumonia or chronic bronchitis in the elderly.

The usefulness of tetracyclines has decreased as a result of the increasing bacterial resistance. In addition, tetracyclines as a group exacerbate renal failure and should not be given to patients with underlying renal disease or with renal impairment associated with extreme old age. A further problem is that the absorption of tetracycline is decreased by calcium, iron, and magnesium salts and by milk and antacids; it should not be prescribed with these compounds frequently taken by the elderly. For these reasons the tetracyclines should not be used in old age. The long-acting tetracycline doxycycline is not nephrotoxic, but its once daily dosage makes it unsuitable for the treatment of bronchopneumonia.

Approximately 10% of penicillin-sensitive patients have hypersensitivity reactions when prescribed cephalosporins. The first-generation cephalosporins are known to cause renal tubular necrosis, particularly in higher dosages and particularly in patients who have already been prescribed loop diuretics prior to commencement of their antibiotic. With the exception of cephadrine, which is not nephrotoxic, these should not be used in old age. Second- and third-generation agents are less nephrotoxic but can only be given parenterally. They should therefore be reserved for particularly severe infection.

Chronic Obstructive Airways Disease

Diagnostic Considerations

Chronic bronchitis and pulmonary emphysema are so intimately related in so many ways that they should always be considered together. However, not all patients with chronic bronchitis have emphysema, and not all emphysema is caused by previous chronic bronchitis. Asthma is a separate entity and should be treated as such.

A patient who develops an acute exacerbation of chronic obstructive airways disease is most commonly infected by *Haemophilus influenzae* and to a lesser extent *Streptococcus pneumoniae*. *Haemophilus* is found as a commensal in the upper respiratory tract, but in favourable circumstances it can invade the lower respiratory tract, producing mucosal inflammation.

Management

Management of chronic bronchitis is often difficult and unrewarding, particularly in old age, where the disease is often more severe and the patient more debilitated than his younger counterpart. Treatment is based on reducing the frequency of the acute exacerbations by treating them with antibiotics, bronchodilators, and oxygen. The frequency of the acute exacerbations can be reduced by encouraging the patient to stop cigarette smoking and seeking or initiating treatment for any increase in sputum production. During influenza epidemics patients should be given an appropriate influenza vaccine. Long-term prophylactic antibiotic therapy also can be very effective in reducing the relapse rate.

Antibiotics

The mainstay of treatment in chronic bronchitis and emphysema is to use appropriate antibiotics in an acute exacerbation. The patient must be trained to recognise the significance of increased sputum production so that early and appropriate antibiotic therapy can be instigated. Amoxycillin or ampicillin in a dose of 250 mg eight-hourly is usually effective.

Until recently doxycycline was a useful alternative, but a recent increase in resistance to it means that it often is ineffective now. Co-trimoxazole should be reserved for unresponsive infections or for patients allergic to ampicillin and amoxycillin.

The sputum should be cultured if a patient fails to respond to the initial antibiotic. In some cases less commonly used antibiotics, including chloramphenicol, may be required for treatment of infections in the elderly patient. Here their high toxicity has to be weighed against their potential benefit.

Bronchodilators

Treatment of bronchospasm is of prime importance, particularly in the patient with limited respiratory reserve. This can be achieved by a variety of agents which include the beta$_2$ stimulators, anticholinergics, xanthine derivatives, and corticosteroids.

Beta$_2$ stimulating drugs such as salbutamol can be used orally, in nebulized form, and by intravenous injection in attempts to achieve maximal bronchodilation. The nebulized form has the least side-effects, apparently because the dosage can be more finely adjusted and not because of any preferential local effect on the airways. Physically and mentally, frail old people experience difficulty in using nebulisers. This should be tackled by painstaking and intensive training. Some drug companies have issued airways for attachment to inhalers so that coordination of pressing the inhaler and inhaling becomes less crucial. There is little difference between the individual beta$_2$ stimulant drugs in terms of efficacy and specificity, although many claims have been made for the individual compounds.

Their side-effects though common are usually minor. They include a fine muscular tremor, and a few patients experience headaches. Palpitations are common, but more severe cardiovascular effects only appear with high dosages or with rapid administration. Both of these should be avoided in the elderly patient. Salbutamol also may increase the blood glucose concentration, a side-effect important in old age where carbohydrate tolerance is already compromised. Coincidental diseases in which beta$_2$ stimulants may cause problems include diabetes, hyperthyroidism, and cardiovascular disorders. A final point is that around 50% of the dose is excreted by the kidney, so that the dose should be adjusted in old people with impaired renal function.

Ipratropium bromide, a local anticholinergic agent has a bronchodilator efficacy similar to that of beta$_2$ receptor agonists. If used in combination with these there is an additional effect greater than that for each individual drug. There is the theoretical risk of a "drying effect" resulting in airways becoming blocked with viscous secretion. In clinical practice, however, the bronchodilator effect is the dominant one. Only if substantial overdosage occurs do generalised anticholinergic effects appear.

Theophylline drugs, particularly theophylline itself and aminophylline, have gained increasing popularity in the last few years as newer preparations have become available for oral administration. Even when such formulations are used, however, theophylline and aminophylline, given orally, still have variable absorption dependent on factors including body weight, age, and heart disease and other pathological conditions. This makes it difficult to calculate the correct dose for old people. It is important therefore to have facilities for monitoring blood levels if the patient is to derive maximum benefit from this treatment. Where this is not practicable, frequent adjustment of dosage may be necessary to achieve maximum bronchodilation with minimum toxicity.

Side-effects from theophylline compounds are common, and include nausea and vomiting, gastro-intestinal irritation, nervousness, dizziness, palpitations, and, occasionally, convulsions. Patients with long-standing underlying ischaemic heart disease, particularly when complicated by arrhythmias, should not be prescribed theophylline and related compounds, as they can precipitate severe and life-threatening arrhythmias.

Particular care also should be taken when giving intravenous aminophylline to old people. While it can be extremely effective in an emergency, serious cardiotoxicity including hypotension, cardiac arrhythmias, and ventricular fibrillation is common. The maximal initial dose should be 250 mg given over a period of not less than 15 min.

Corticosteroid Therapy

Studies of the effect of corticosteroid therapy on acute exacerbations of chronic obstructive airways disease have shown that there is a marked improvement in terms of morbidity and mortality in patients given steroid therapy as compared to those given placebo. It is important, however, that treatment be tailed off rapidly after remission of the exacerbation. In old people corticosteroids should only be used if other measures have failed to control the exacerbation. Long-term low-dose corticosteroids may improve respiratory function, but produce a wide range of serious side-effects in old people.

Bronchial Asthma

Though much less common than in young people, bronchial asthma can occur for the first time in old age and should be treated in the same manner as in younger individuals using conventional therapy (Burr et al. 1979). However, old people often have both impaired lung function and a degree of irreversible lung disease, which may need treatment after remission of the acute episode.

Tuberculosis

Diagnostic Considerations

Tuberculosis is less common than it was in former years, but there still is a large reservoir of disease in the elderly which all too frequently goes unrecognised (Iseman 1980). About 10%–25% of old people have evidence of healed (dormant) infection and therefore the recurrence of infection is a constant threat. This often is accentuated by diabetes, malignancy, or cortico-steroid therapy. Both the clinical and radiological presentations of tuberculosis in old age can be quite atypical. Reaction to the tuberculin test may be suppressed, often as a result of subnutrition or chronic ill health.

Old people in residential care and in nursing homes are particularly at risk. Several studies have shown that if tuberculin tests are performed on all patients admitted over several years, and rechecked annually thereafter, there is a two- to threefold increase in the proportion of persons who react positively. It is advisable therefore that a resident with a positive tuberculin test at the time of admission to a nursing home should have an X-ray to exclude active disease. This should decrease the risk of spread amongst the residents.

The diagnosis of tuberculosis is best confirmed by examination of the sputum for acid and alcohol fast bacilli using direct microscopy. Specimens also should be cultured for sensitivity to specific antituberculin drugs. Treatment, however, should not await these results. A delay of 2 months is likely to be fatal, particularly in an elderly patient debilitated from other diseases. If sputum cannot be obtained, laryngeal swabs and gastric wash-outs, obtained upon waking in the morning, are useful substitutes. Lung or pleural biopsy may be indicated in a few individual cases.

Management

An elderly patient should be admitted to hospital for the initiation of antituberculous therapy, particularly if the tuberculosis is associated with other diseases. Whilst previously it was felt that the best results were achieved by using double drug therapy for a period of 18–24 months, recently developed bactericidal drugs such as rifampicin and isoniazid have reduced the period required for effective control to only 9 months.

Following discharge from hospital, very carefuly checks need to be kept on the old people. Those with mental impairment may mismanage their medication with disastrous results, either due to side-effects from overdosage, or recurrence of the pulmonary tuberculosis from omission of doses.

The agents most commonly used in the United Kingdom and France are isoniazid and rifampicin given once daily for 9 months and supplemented for the initial 8–12 weeks with ethambutol. Some workers argue that there is little benefit from the addition of the third drug. However, though it adds to the cost and toxicity of treatment, it provides important protection against any resistant organisms which may be present. Individual drugs used in tuberculosis and their relative risks are outlined below.

Isoniazid.   The major side-effect of isoniazid is a peripheral neuropathy. This is the result of drug-induced pyridoxine deficiency, and is dose-dependent. It has become much rarer since the routine addition of pyridoxine in doses of 50–300 mg/day to isoniazid therapy. Old people who are alcoholic, diabetic, or epileptic are at additional risk of developing a neuropathy. Isoniazid also occasionally may cause liver damage. It is uncertain whether this is toxic or allergic in origin. Symptoms usually occur within 6–8 weeks of commencing therapy and are particularly common when other antituberculous agents are used along with isoniazid. These include rifampicin or para-aminosalicylic acid. If isoniazid is stopped, the prognosis for the resolution of liver damage usually is good.

Rifampicin.   In spite of a formidable list of possible adverse reactions, severe side-effects are extremely rare (Table 5.2). Usually the only manifestation of liver damage is a transient elevation of enzymes, but icterus occurs occasionally, particularly if the drug is used in combination with isoniazid. Increased hepatic enzyme induction may reduce blood and tissue concentrations of other drugs, such as the coumarin anticoagulants. A beneficial side-effect of rifampicin is that it turns the colour of urine orange or red. This is useful in establishing the compliance of elderly patients who may forget to take the medication.

Table 5.2. Adverse effects of rifampicin

Anorexia and nausea

Transient increase in SGOT and SGPT levels
  (particularly when given with isoniazid)

Hypersensitivity reaction—exanthema, pyrexia,
  shock, haemolysis, leucopenia, and
  thrombocytopenia

Hepatic enzyme inductions

Clearly, rifampicin should be used with care in patients with pre-existing liver or renal damage, or if other hepatotoxic drugs are administered simultaneously. A previous history of drug allergy increases the risk of a patient developing an allergic reaction to rifampicin.

Ethambutol.   Ethambutol is effective against tuberculous bacteria and atypical mycobacteria by blocking nucleic acid synthesis. It often is used in combination with other antituberculous agents for the first 8–12 weeks. Dosage has to be adapted to renal function.

Its most important side-effects are diminution of visual acuity and colour vision. These ocular effects are dose-dependent, with irreversible changes occurring at higher levels. Pre-existing liver damage and diabetic changes in the fundus of the eye increase the risk of these. As soon as the patient complains of visual disturbance, the drug should be stopped. This is even more urgent if an examination of the eyes confirms the adverse reaction.

Streptomycin.   Streptomycin is an aminoglycoside. Major side-effects, particularly in the elderly, are those of ototoxicity and renal damage. Ototoxicity is particularly common in old people who have impaired renal function or who also are on potent diuretics like frusemide. Streptomycin should not be used in the elderly unless sensitivity tests indicate that there is no alternative. Administration should be monitored closely, with particular reference to the drug's well defined side-effects.

Para-aminosalicylic Acid.   Para-aminosalicylic acid should seldom be used now because of side-effects, which include gastro-intestinal irritation. These are particularly common in the elderly.

References

Barker WH, Mullooly JP (1980) Influenza vaccination of elderly persons. JAMA 244: 2547–2549

Burr ML, Charles TJ, Roy K, Seaton A (1979) Asthma in the elderly: an epidemiological survey. Br Med J 1: 1041–1044

Caird FI, Akhtar AJ (1972) Chronic respiratory disease in the elderly. Thorax 27: 764–768

Iseman MD (1980) Tuberculosis in the elderly: treating the "white plague". Geriatrics 35 (March): 90–107

Milne JS, Williamson J (1972) Respiratory function tests in older people. Clin Sci 42: 371–381

6 Disorders of the Alimentary System

Hiatus Hernia

Well over half of old people are likely to have a hiatus hernia (Fig. 6.1). This means that before treatment is instituted the physician should make certain that the symptoms in question are related to the hernia. Chest pain may be due to coronary artery disease, flatulence due to gallstones, and anaemia resulting from duodenal ulcer or a carcinoma of the bowel. Again the hernia may not be causing any symptoms, so that drug treatment is inappropriate. If the pain is related to a hernia it only occurs if there is oesophagitis.

If the condition is causing symptoms, the patient should be given advice on his posture, habits, and diet (Table 6.1). Along with this advice, he should be given antacids and should take these between meals when there are symptoms, after meals, and before bedtime. Antacids may be given along with alginic acid (Gaviscon) so that they form a viscous solution, floating on the surface of gastric acid, thus forming a barrier between acid and the oesophageal mucosa. Clinical trials, however, suggest that this combination is no more effective than a simple antacid.

Table 6.1. Advice for patient with hiatus hernia on posture, habits, and diet (Richter and Castell 1981)

1. Eat last meal several hours before going to bed
2. Avoid lying down after meals
3. Elevate head of the bed by six inches
4. Reduce weight if obese
5. Avoid tight garments
6. Avoid fat, chocolate, citrus juices, or peppermint
7. Avoid alcohol
8. Avoid smoking

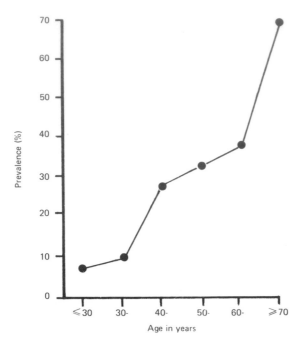

Fig. 6.1. Prevalence of hiatus hernia in subjects receiving a barium meal and swallow for abdominal pain (Priddie 1966).

Most patients respond to a regime which embodies postural and dietary advice, and the administration of adequate quantities of antacids. If they do not, cimetidine or ranitidine should be added. These act by blocking the H_2 receptors thus reducing acid secretion. They often produce rapid symptomatic relief, and evidence is mounting that the inflammatory changes of oesophagitis may also be reversed. The recommended dosage of cimetidine is 800–1000 mg daily and for ranitidine 300 mg daily. Cimetidine may cause some confusion in an elderly patient, particularly if he has renal impairment or when it is used with benzodiazepines. Ranitidine may be safer in this context and has been shown to be as effective in relieving the symptoms of oesophagitis.

An alternative is to block acid reflux by increasing pressure at the gastro-oesophageal sphincter and improving peristaltic activity within the oesophagus. Bethanechol has this dual effect and in a dose of 25 mg four times daily reduces heartburn. It can be given along with cimetidine. However, large doses can cause mental confusion and urinary retention, so that in old people with multiple pathology it probably is safer to reserve it for patients who fail to respond to the H_2 antagonists and antacids alone. Metoclopramide also modifies oesophageal motility, but there is little evidence of efficacy in controlling symptoms of gastro-oesophageal reflux.

In old age one of the more common complications of oesophagitis is that it may cause benign strictures. Bougienage is the mainstay of management, but this may have to be performed at frequent intervals in frail and anxious individuals. Repeated bougienage also carries with it a small but significant risk of rupturing the oesophagus. Old people thus may have to be left until the condition is producing severe dysphagia, and they have lost a considerable amount of weight. It was hoped that the H_2 antagonists might reduce the rate at which restenosis occurred. As yet, however, the case for its use in stenosis remains "not proven".

Peptic Ulcers

Autopsy studies have shown that in men duodenal ulcers reach a peak prevalence in middle age, which falls off in old age (Fig. 6.2). Gastric ulcers, though less common, show a similar pattern. In women, duodenal ulcers, though less common than in men, reach a peak prevalence in middle age which is maintained into old age (Fig. 6.3). The prevalence of gastric ulcers rises with increasing age to equal that of duodenal ulcers in old age. The decline of peptic ulceration in old age for men might be explained by decline in gastric acidity with age. The increased prevalence of peptic ulcers in old women might represent removal of the protective effects of oestrogens, so that ulcers become almost as common as in old men.

There are no firm data on the proportion of peptic ulcers giving rise to symptoms in old age, but clinical experience suggests that typical dyspeptic

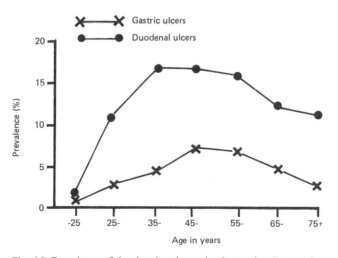

Fig. 6.2. Prevalence of duodenal and gastric ulcers related to age in men (Watkinson 1960).

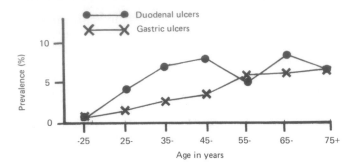

Fig. 6.3. Prevalence of duodenal and gastric ulcers related to age in women (Watkinson 1960).

symptoms are often absent. The presentation may be that of non-specific weight loss, iron-deficiency anaemia, or even mental confusion. Reasons for this may include an increased threshold for deep pain, an impaired immunological response to trauma and a reduction in acid secretion. This means that, in treating peptic ulcers in the elderly, doctors are often involved in managing disorders such as weight loss, vomiting, anaemia, or confusion rather than controlling epigastric pain. Ulcer healing rather than mere pain relief thus may be their priority more often than in younger patients.

Antacids

Antacids are only marginally better than placebo in relieving pain associated with peptic ulceration. If used for this purpose an antacid should be given in a dose of 15–30 ml half an hour before meals and at bedtime. In old people a magnesium preparation such as magnesium trisilicate mixture is preferable to an aluminium one, in that it will have a laxative rather than a constipating effect.

Antacids are of proven value in healing peptic ulcers. Unfortunately, the dose necessary for this is 30 ml of liquid antacid 1 and 3 h after meals and before bed, giving a daily dose of 210 ml. This regime is unlikely to be acceptable to most physically and mentally frail old people.

The H₂ Antagonists

Cimetidine and ranitidine reduce gastric acid secretion by blocking the H_2 histamine receptors in the gastric mucosa. They heal 65%–90% of duodenal ulcers in 4–6 weeks. Though they are also effective against gastric ulcers, the healing rates are poorer. The recommended doses are 200 mg three times daily with 400 mg at bedtime for cimetidine and 150 mg twice daily for ranitidine for

6 weeks. Relapse often follows discontinuation, so that a maintenance dose of 400 mg cimetidine or 150 mg of ranitidine at bedtime may be necessary.

Used in short courses, the drugs have a low toxicity. Episodes of mental confusion occasionally have been reported, particularly with cimetidine, but most old people tolerate the H_2 antagonists well. Rare cases of gynaecomastia or galactorrhoea are of academic interest rather than of major clinical importance. Hepatic dysfunction manifested by rising serum transaminase concentrations rarely causes difficulty. Suppression of hepatic microsomal oxidation is more relevant in that old people on propranolol or coumarin anticoagulants may develop toxic levels of these when treated subsequently with cimetidine, but apparently not with ranitidine.

The long-term effects of the drugs are uncertain. They suppress intrinsic factor secretion and this could be important in old age where gastric secretion already is compromised. Again, T-lymphocytes have H_2 receptors, and suppression of lymphocyte function could be disastrous in old age where immunological surveillance is already disturbed. Fortunately, a detailed investigation failed to establish such an effect (MacGregor et al. 1977). Finally, there is speculation that the H_2 antagonists might result in the conversion of nitroso-compounds into carcinogenic agents in the stomach. There is no supporting evidence for this. Even if there was, it is unlikely that most elderly patients would survive long enough for their gastric mucosa to undergo malignant change. A much greater danger is that a malignant ulcer might be treated inappropriately with H_2 antagonists. This must be recognised when in a frail old patient the hazards and discomforts of endoscopy and contrast radiography are being balanced against the dangers of empirical treatment with an H_2 antagonist.

Carbenoxolone

This liquorice derivative is particularly effective in the healing of gastric ulcers. It also has potent mineralocorticoid effects causing salt and water retention and potassium depletion. Since many old people have hypertension or congestive cardiac failure, and their stores of potassium are low already, they should never be given carbenoxolone. Caved-(S) (deglycyrrhizined liquorice extract) has less of a salt-retaining effect and therefore may be of benefit in some patients in whom carbenoxolone is contraindicated.

Colloidal Bismuth Compounds

Tri-potassium dicitrato bismuthate (De-Nol) reacts with gastric juices to form a protein bismuthate which coats and protects an ulcer crater. Over 4–6 weeks it heals 78%–90% of duodenal, and 85%–90% of gastric ulcers. Dosage is 5 ml dissolved in 20 ml water three times a day at least half an hour before meals and at bedtime. This is now available in tablet form for patients who find it unpalatable in the liquid form. Its ammoniacal odour is unimportant in anosmic old people, while black discoloration of the stool is a problem for the doctor and not the patient. In view of its efficacy and low toxicity, De-Nol is the drug of choice for gastric ulcers in the elderly.

Sucrolfate

This sulphated polysaccharide is little used in Britain. It is effective in both duodenal and gastric ulcers, however, and has a low toxicity. A marginal disadvantage for old people is that it causes constipation in up to 10% of subjects.

Recently developed agents, then, have revolutionised the management of peptic ulcers in the elderly. They should only be used, however, where the site and nature of the ulcer has been adequately investigated. There may be the temptation simply to put an 85-year-old woman with abdominal pain on cimetidine or De-Nol. To do so is to run the risk of mismanaging anything from constipation through cholecystitis to gastric carcinoma.

Biliary Disorders

The prevalence of gallstones rises with age so that almost half of women and over a quarter of men over 90 years have this condition (Fig. 6.4). In many of these patients gallstones are asymptomatic. If left, however, there is some risk that they will cause symptoms, or indeed result in a complication such as bile duct obstruction or carcinoma of the gallbladder. However, even in healthy young people where the operative mortality is less than 1% and the risk of bile duct stenosis or failure to remove all stones less than 2.5%, the case for surgery is doubtful. In old age the high prevalence of gallstones alone would make surgery on all cases logistically impossible. Furthermore, old people with asymptomatic stones may not live long enough to develop symptoms or complications. Finally, though old age itself is not a contraindication to surgery, patients with multiple pathology obviously have an increased operative mortality. In old age, then, surgery should not be undertaken in patients with no symptoms. It should be considerd only for patients who have had one or more episodes of acute cholecystitis. Contraindications include chronic mental impairment likely to be made worse by an operation and anaesthetic; severe systemic disease such as congestive cardiac failure certain to produce a high mortality; and extreme old age (i.e. over 90), where the patient may not surive long enough to have a recurrent attack or develop complications.

If surgery is contraindicated, medical treatment should be considered. The most effective agents are the bile salt chenodeoxycholic acid and the synthetic agent ursodeoxycholic acid. Given orally they are absorbed from the gut and excreted by the liver into the biliary tract. At this site, chenodeoxycholic acid assists increased concentration and helps prevent cholesterol from crystallising

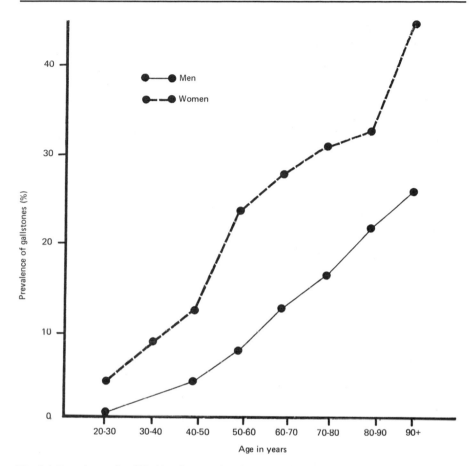

Fig. 6.4. Prevalence of gallbladder disease related to age (Lieber 1952).

out to form cholesterol stones. Further effects arc that it tends to decrease the hepatic secretion and the dietary intake of cholesterol. Care should be taken to limit its use to situations in which it is likely to be effective (Table 6.2). Where the preconditions are met, dissolution of stones is effective in 80% of cases but, dependent on stone size, the process will take between 6 months and 2 years. The starting oral dose should be 1000 mg daily. This may have to be reduced if there are side-effects, but a lower dose delays stone dissolution.

The main side-effect is diarrhoea, occurring in up to 50% of patients. This is the result of unabsorbed chenodeoxycholic acid acting as an osmotic laxative in the colon. With time, colonic mucosal cells adapt to the situation, so that less water is excreted and more reabsorbed through them. Diarrhoea, thus, tends to be a temporary phenomenon responding to a temporary reduction of dosage and adapting to a later increase to original levels. The newer synthetic agent,

Table 6.2. Situations in which the use of chenodeoxycholic acid or ursodeoxycholic acid is likely to be effective

1. Gallstones should be made up of cholesterol
2. Gallstones should be radiotranslucent
3. Gallstones should be less than 2 cm in diameter
4. The gallbladder should be functioning normally
5. Gallstones should not be obstructing the common bile duct
6. Liver function tests should be normal

ursodeoxycholic acid, does not have this effect of producing diarrhoea; it is as effective as chenodeoxycholic acid in producing gallstone dissolution and is now the drug of choice for the medical treatment of gallstones.

The risk of gallstone complications does not disappear until the stones are dissolved completely. Patients thus should be kept under close review with a cholecystogram being repeated once every 6 months. In old people, ursodeoxycholic acid probably should be continued indefinitely, since cessation of therapy is associated with a high recurrence rate.

Only 40% of patients with gallstones are suitable for treatment with ursodeoxycholic acid. The remainder should be left untreated if asymptomatic. In those with symptoms, clinicians, in coming to a decision about surgery, have to balance the risk of a high mortality associated with an attack of cholecystitis against the high mortality accompanying elective cholecystectomy in mentally or physically frail elderly patients.

Cholestatic Jaundice

Table 6.3 lists the more common causes of jaundice in elderly patients admitted to hospital. That drug-induced cholestasis figures prominently in this is a reflection of the large number of potentially hepatotoxic drugs used in old

Table 6.3. Causes of jaundice in elderly patients admitted to hospital (Eastwood 1971)

Cancer involving bile tract	22%
Drugs	21%
Calculi in bile tract	16%
Hepatitis	15%
Hepatic secondaries	12%
Cirrhosis	10%
Haemolysis	5%

people. In many instances toxicity is related to a hypersensitivity reaction in which the drug acts as a hapten. This causes infiltration of the portal zones with lymphocytes, plasma cells, and eosinophils, accompanied by blockage of bile canaliculi. The condition usually resolves when the offending drug is stopped. Table 6.4 lists drugs commonly used in old people which may cause cholestatic jaundice.

Table 6.4. Drugs commonly used in old people causing cholestatic jaundice (Davies 1977)

Cause jaundice frequently	Cause jaundice occasionally	Cause jaundice rarely
Chlorpromazine (2%–5%)	Other phenothiazines	Tolbutamide
Rifampicin	Chlorpropamide	Chlordiazepoxide
Isoniazid	Sodium aurithomaleate	Diazepam
PAS	Tricyclic antidepressants	Phenobarbitone
Erythromycin	Phenytoin	Allopurinol
	Phenylbutazone	Penicillin
	Sulphonamides	Ampicillin
	Co-trimoxazole	
	Nitrofurantoin	
	Hydralazine	

Chronic Active Hepatitis

This is a condition characterised by a round cell infiltration of liver portal tracts in which infiltrations from neighbouring tracts coalesce and so progressively destroy the normal liver architecture. The clinical picture is that of vague lassitude sometimes accompanied by mild jaundice. Serum concentrations of bilirubin, alkaline phosphatase, and transaminase usually are elevated. The condition, though originally described in young women, also occurs in old age. As with many other disorders in old age, it may present as mental impairment, possibly due to a hepatic encephalopathy.

Serum from patients may or may not contain hepatitis B antigen, and patients without the antigen respond well to corticosteroids. The elderly do equally well on treatment. This, however, should be reserved for patients with clinical symptoms and signs. It confers no benefit on those who merely have abnormal liver function tests. This is relevant in old age where the side-effects of corticosteroids are particularly serious (Chap. 8). In older people, indeed, there is particular merit in combining corticosteroids with the antimitotic agent azathioprine. A maintenance dose of 10 mg prednisolone and 50 mg azathioprine is just as effective and has fewer side-effects than a larger dose of corticosteroids.

Malabsorption

In the elderly, malabsorption should always be considered as a possible cause of anaemia, bone pain, or chronic diarrhoea. In one series 13 of 33 elderly patients with such disorders had malabsorption as defined by xylose absorption, Dicopac, iron absorption, and faecal fat excretion test (Montgomery et al. 1978). Table 6.5 details the underlying pathologies in a series of patients over 50 presenting with steatorrhoea (Price et al. 1977).

Table 6.5. Causes of steatorrhoea in patients aged over 50 years (Price et al. 1977)

Coeliac disease		16%
Pancreatic insufficiency		14%
Postgastrectomy		8%
Jejunal diverticula		2%
Tropical spore		2%
Others		5%
	Total	47%

When coeliac disease is encountered in old age, consideration should be given to the high cost and inconvenience of a gluten-free diet. It may be more appropriate to leave the primary pathology untreated and to treat with folic acid, vitamin D, calcium, and iron supplements as necessary. Chronic pancreatitis again should be treated with vitamin and mineral supplements, including vitamin K. Absorption can be improved by giving pancreatin, a powder containing protease, amylase, and lipase. The amount given varies between 2 and 8 g daily in divided doses, dependent on change in faecal fat excretion. Since it is destroyed by acid, it is recommended that acid secretion be suppressed with cimetidine. This is not necessary in old people with atrophic gastritis. A pentagastrin test meal should always be performed before resorting to a drug whose long-term effects are uncertain.

Malabsorption often develops for the first time in old age many years after gastric surgery. Treatment consists of giving iron, cyanocobalamin, vitamin D, and calcium supplements. Extra protein may be given as skimmed milk, but old people often dislike high-protein diets and there may be difficulty in ensuring compliance.

Malabsorption due to colonisation of the gut from bacteria in duodenal or jejunal diverticula should be treated with mineral and vitamin supplements—cyanocobalamin and folic acid are often particularly deficient due to utilisation by bacteria. Infection should be cleared using a broad-spectrum antibiotic. The tetracyclines are effective, but are potentially nephrotoxic in old people with renal impairment. Here, the drug of choice is doxycycline, a tetracycline with no renal effects. A further advantage is that the 100-mg dose need only be given once daily.

Old people suffering from chronic inflammatory or malignant disorders also may have some degree of malabsorption. Examples include rheumatoid arthritis and carcinomatosis. Here treatment consists of mineral and vitamin supplements, combined with management, if possible, of the underlying condition.

Disorders of the Large Bowel

Diverticular Disease

Diverticular disease of the colon develops late in life and over the age of 80 it affects more than 40% of subjects (Figure 6.5). Presenting symptoms include constipation, diarrhoea, melaena, nausea, vomiting, heartburn, flatulence, frequency, and dysuria. Since both these symptoms and diverticular disease are very common in old people it is important to make sure that symptoms and

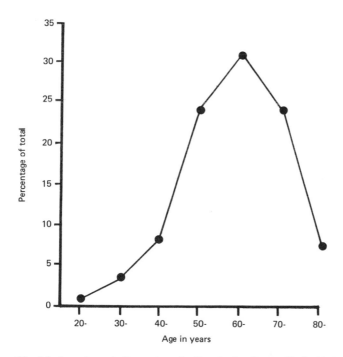

Fig. 6.5. Age of onset of symptoms in diverticular disease (Parks 1969).

...iological changes really are linked together before embarking on a prolonged course of treatment.

The first essential is to increase bulk in the diet by using bran in a starting dose of two teaspoonsful three times per day, reducing this if it causes flatulence, distension, or watery stools. If this fails to control symptoms, a smooth muscle relaxant such as alverine citrate 60 mg three times daily or mebeverine 135 mg three times daily should be used. Drugs relaxing smooth muscle by depression of parasympathetic activity should be avoided. If the disease is associated with a paracolic abscess, an appropriate antibiotic should be used.

Ulcerative Colitis and Crohn's Disease

Though most common in youth and middle age, ulcerative colitis can occur for the first time in old age (Fig. 6.6). When starting treatment it is important to ensure that an accurate diagnosis has been made. The incidence of Crohn's disease rises with advancing years, so that in old age it is, in fact, more common

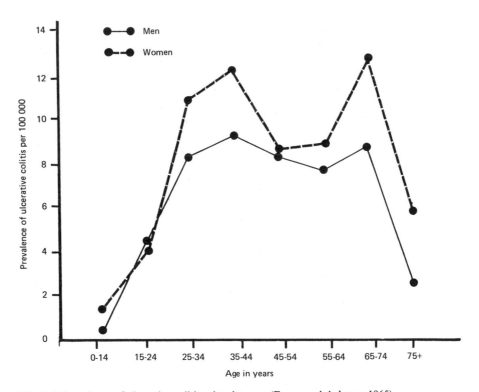

Fig. 6.6. Prevalence of ulcerative colitis related to age (Evans and Acheson 1965).

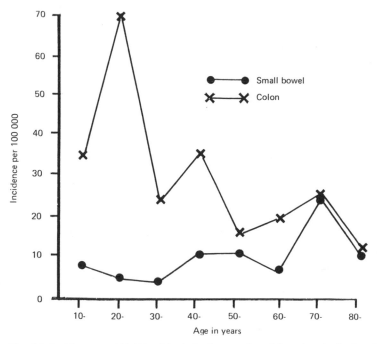

Fig. 6.7. Incidence per 100 000 of Crohn's disease of small bowel and of colon (Kyle 1971).

than ulcerative colitis (Fig. 6.7). Another condition presenting with a similar clinical picture is ischaemic colitis.

An exacerbation of ulcerative colitis should be treated with up to 40 mg prednisolone daily, and 100-mg enemas of hydrocortisone sodium succinate twice daily dependent upon the severity of symptoms. Maintenance therapy consists of sulphasalazine, a minimum of 2 g daily. Less information is available on the treatment of choice in an exacerbation of Crohn's colitis, but it seems likely that either corticosteroids or sulphasalazine can be used with benefit.

When ulcerative colitis occurs for the first time in an elderly patient, the risks of it persisting long enough to produce malignancy are low, so that surgery should be reserved for patients with toxic megacolon. There is a high rate of recurrence after surgery for Crohn's disease of the colon so that, here again, it should be offered only to patients with toxic megacolon.

Ischaemic Colitis

Ischaemic colitis classically presents in the elderly with sharp left iliac fossa pain, progressing to generalised abdominal pain associated with the passage of a small motion mixed with dark blood or clots.

...emic colitis has three outcomes: progression to gangrene (which is, ...unately, infrequent), resolution, or stricture formation. Diagnosis is usually ...made on the basis of a straight abdominal X-ray where thumb printing may be seen, or either barium enema or colonoscopy.

Treatment is conservative with a combination of bed-rest, intravenous fluid repletion, and systemic antibiotics (e.g. a combination of ampicillin, gentamycin, and metronidazole). Systemic antibiotics are said to reduce the frequency of dangerous sequelae.

Constipation

In healthy old people there is no change in the frequency of bowel motions with increasing age. If such individuals are concerned about bowel function they should be encouraged to take regular physical exercise; to obey a call to stool when it occurs; to attempt to pass a motion at a regular time each day, preferably after a meal; and to increase the fibre content of their diet. Ways of doing this include switching from white to wholemeal bread, and regularly taking breakfast cereals, preferably such ones as All-bran and Shredded Wheat.

Old people with limited mobility are more likely to be constipated. They do not take sufficient exercise to stimulate colonic activity, they often fail to respond to a call for defaecation, and weakness of the abdominal and pelvic muscles makes defaecation more difficult. Once this pattern is established, faeces lie longer in the colon, becoming increasingly dehydrated and hard and thus more difficult to pass.

The most effective way of preventing such a pattern from developing is to put a patient on regular doses of bran. A dose of 10 g twice daily taken with meals increases both the wet and dry weight of stools, and enhances the excretion of bile acids, fat, and electrolytes. Taken in too large a dose, bran causes flatulence and abdominal distension, but this can easily be remedied by reducing dosage. Patients may prefer to take bran in tablet form, for which proprietary preparations such as Fybranta and Proctofibe are available. Others who dislike bran may prefer the bulk-forming drug ispaghula husk taken as Fybogel, Isogel, or Metamucil. This is just as effective as bran and has the same range of side-effects.

Though both bran and ispaghula are excellent laxatives it must be recognised that many people dislike their taste, so that considerable reinforcement and supervision may be required to ensure that, outside hospital, patients do not revert to more traditional forms of therapy.

Another way of increasing stool bulk is to increase its water content by using an osmotic purgative. Lactulose is a fructose-lactose disaccharide which is split into its monosaccharide components by organisms in the colon. This increases the osmotic pressure within the colon, thus increasing its fluid content. Unfortunately, bacteria react with lactulose to produce large quantities of gas. Patients thus often have severe abdominal distension, borborygmi, colic, and flatulence. These side-effects are much more prominent than with bran or ispaghula, and restrict the use of lactulose largely to patients with portal systemic encephalopathy. Here the effect of lactulose in reducing ammonia absorption is important.

A wide range of laxatives acting by means of a stimulant effect on the colon are available. They include the anthracene glycosides senna and cascara and the diphenylmethane derivatives bisacodyl and sodium picosulphate. All these agents are effective in the short-term treatment of episodes of constipation in otherwise healthy old people. When used over prolonged periods, however, they may induce tolerance, and even cause myenteric plexus damage (see section entitled "Laxative Abuse" below). They should not be used, therefore, as a substitute for bulk laxatives.

Many patients have dry and hard stools and benefit from a stool-softening agent. The traditional one was liquid paraffin. This mixes incompletely with water and faeces and unmixed paraffin often leaks from the anus. Again, it dissolves fat-soluble vitamins, so that it accentuates vitamin D deficiency in old people. Finally, patients with dysphagia or gastro-oesophageal reflux aspirate paraffin so that they have recurrent bouts of pneumonia and develop extensive pulmonary fibrosis. Liquid paraffin, therefore, should not be given to old people.

Dioctyl sodium sulphosuccinate is the agent of choice. This is a detergent which mixes with and softens faeces. Dosage is 37.5–200 mg daily in divided doses. Though it can damage the gastric mucosa, there are no reports of this having serious clinical effects. However, it should be used with care in patients with ascorbic acid deficiency, or in those on gastric irritants such as aspirin, indomethacin, or phenylbutazone.

Faecal Impaction

Old people often are admitted to hospital with a colon loaded with hard faeces. This causes a wide range of problems including restlessness and confusion, urinary incontinence, and the leakage of liquid around the hard mass from the proximal part of the colon. Under normal circumstances faeces moving into the rectum are evacuated by peristaltic and skeletal muscle activity. Sick old people, however, may be too weak to respond to this reflex so that antiperistaltic activity moves the faeces back into the sigmoid colon where they become progressively more dehydrated. At this stage, bulk or irritant laxatives only add to the mass of faeces in the colon and accentuate spurious diarrhoea.

A more rational approach is to give an enema to expand the rectum and thus stimulate peristalsis and evacuation. Fletcher's phosphate enema is a hypertonic solution which takes up water into the colon from surrounding tissues. Each enema contains 120 ml fluid. If the colon is to be cleared of faeces this will have to be given daily for 7–10 days. After this the patient can go on to a bulk laxative, adding a stool-softening agent if necessary.

If the patient remains immobile, bulk laxatives may be ineffective and merely add to the mass of faeces in the colon. In such circumstances a better approach is to continue with a stool softener, but avoid a bulk laxative and give a phosphate enema once a week.

The old soap and water enema should be consigned to history. It has a low osmotic pressure, so that large quantities are absorbed from the colon into the circulation where they cause haemodilution and circulatory collapse.

As an alternative to daily enemas, faecal stasis may be treated with whole gut irrigation. The technique involves passing a nasogastric tube and giving both frusemide 40 mg and metoclopramide 10 mg intravenously. Isotonic saline at body temperature is then infused down the tube at a rate of 2.5–3 l/h, while the patient is seated on a rubber ring over a commode in a warm, secluded, and well ventilated room. The process is continued until the rectal discharge is clear. It is difficult to make a value judgement on whether this rapid but drastic attack on an impaction is preferable to a prolonged and rather degrading treatment with daily enemas. Consideration also has to be given to the risk of a saline infusion precipitating congestive cardiac failure in a susceptible individual.

Laxative Abuse

In old age, concern about constipation is as great a problem as the condition itself. Evidence of this is the increased incidence of laxative self-administration with advancing years (Fig. 6.8). A probable reason for this is the medical climate of past generations, which dwelt on the toxic effects of a loaded colon and the health and vigour supposedly associated with an empty one. With continued use irritant laxatives, particularly the anthraquinones, become less and less effective and symptoms of constipation more and more severe.

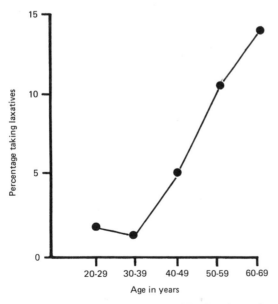

Fig. 6.8. Percentage of population taking laxatives at least once per week (Connell et al. 1965).

In this situation, pathologists have demonstrated mucosal inflammation, hypertrophy of the muscularis mucosa, and thinning of outer muscle layers. Special histological stains show up damage to and destruction of myenteric plexus neurones. There usually is considerable abdominal distension, and there may be characteristic radiological changes, consisting of a dilated colon which has lost its normal haustral and mucosal pattern. Sigmoidoscopy may reveal patchy pigmentation of the colon (melanosis coli).

Treatment consists of substituting the anthraquinone with a high-fibre diet or with a bulk or saline laxative. If this does not work, repeated enemas may be required, but in old people it is doubtful whether the more radical approach of colonic resection can ever be justified.

As with many other disorders, the best way of controlling the inappropriate use of laxatives is to provide the patient with rational advice and treatment at the initial stages of his problem. Bowel regulation is often delegated to the community nurse or to the ward sister, but in old people it is of such major importance that the doctor should be involved at all stages.

Diarrhoea

In frail old people the most common cause of loose liquid motions is a faecal impaction associated with rectal leakage. Treatment involves clearance of the underlying impaction. The administration of codeine or loperamide will make the condition worse.

Bowel infections are also common (Fig. 6.9). Many episodes of diarrhoea in which a cause has not been identified probably are related to undiagnosed rickettsial or viral infections. Usually the condition is treated merely symptomatically using absorbent materials or drugs reducing motility. These include codeine phosphate, diphenoxylate hydrochloride, loperamide hydrochloride,

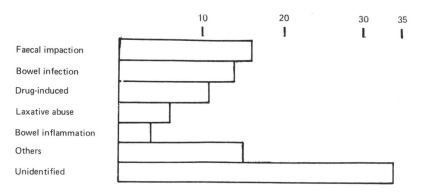

Fig. 6.9. Causes of diarrhoea in 100 patients admitted to hospital with diarrhoea (Pentland and Pennington 1980).

and a kaolin and morphine mixture. In most cases, antibiotics should be avoided (see section entitled "Pseudomembranous Colitis" below).

Old people, by virtue of renal impairment, have great difficulty in adapting to the additional stress of gastro-enteritis, so that they rapidly develop sodium, potassium, or water depletion. Replacement therapy thus is frequently required. This preferably should be given orally. Parenteral fluids should be given with extreme caution, keeping a close watch for peripheral oedema, pulmonary crepitations, and jugular venous congestion. Direct measurement of the central venous pressure also is necessary. Blood urea, serum sodium, and serum potassium concentrations also should be monitored regularly. Even with these precautions, it is alarming how rapidly a susceptible individual can develop hypokalaemia or go into congestive cardiac failure. Every case of diarrhoea in the elderly, therefore, needs to be treated as a potentially serious emergency.

Pseudomembranous Colitis

This is a particularly severe form of enteritis which may follow the oral administration of a wide range of antibiotics. These include ampicillin, co-trimoxazole, tetracycline, penicillin, amoxycillin, lincomycin, clindamycin, and aminoglycosides with or without metronidazole. It is particularly common in frail elderly patients where it is associated with a mucous and watery diarrhoea. Pyrexia and leucocytosis are common, but may be masked by immunological incompetence in old age. Sigmoidoscopy may establish the diagnosis by revealing multiple white plaques adherent to the mucosa. Biopsy reveals inflammation of the submucosa with disruption of the mucosa, ulcers being full of mucin and polymorphs covered with a pseudomembrane of firm mucus and polymorphs. Mortality is high, occurring in 70% of patients aged over 65. The disorder results from the overgrowth of *Clostridium difficile* in circumstances where other bacteria with less antibiotic resistance are cleared from the gut lumen. The organism usually is treated with vancomycin given in an oral dose of 125 mg every 6 h. It also is sensitive, in vitro, to metronidazole, but since this is absorbed from the gut, levels in the colon are very low and relatively ineffective.

Drug-Induced Diarrhoea

Many drugs have a direct irritant effect on the colon. Antibiotics likely to cause diarrhoea in this way include ampicillin, tetracycline, chloramphenicol, linco-mycin, and clindamycin. Co-trimoxazole and the cephalosporins cause gastro-intestinal disturbance less frequently than these others. Other drugs with an irritant effect include the anti-inflammatory analgesics and iron, potassium, or calcium salts. Magnesium salts are poorly absorbed and act as osmotic aperients.

Faecal Incontinence

In old age, faecal incontinence often is due to faecal impaction or diarrhoea. Some patients have a lax anal sphincter or rectal prolapse which can be treated with surgery.

Most forms of faecal incontinence, then, respond to treatment. An exception is faecal incontinence occasionally encountered in gross mental impairment. Here the only way of reducing the severity of the incontinence is to put the patient on codeine, and to clear the colon out once a week with a phosphate enema. It must be emphasised that faecal incontinence is caused by dementia only in exceptional circumstances. In most cases a local factor can be identified and treated.

Other Alimentary Conditions

Carious teeth, worn dentures, reduce salivary secretion, reduced immunological surveillance, and bad habits such as heavy smoking all account for the fact that mouth ulcers and infections are common in old age. Improved dental care and adequate oral hygiene would do much to eliminate these conditions. There are several disorders, however, which require treatment with specific medication.

Aphthous Ulcers

Many people suffer from recurrent crops of greyish-white ulcers with a reddish margin affecting the tongue and buccal mucosa. These can occur at any age, but are particularly prevalent in women after the menopause. Many remedies have been tried, but the only one of proven efficacy is hydrocortisone hemisuccinate. This is prepared as pellets containing 2.5 mg. Patients are instructed to dissolve these in the region of the ulcer, and to take up to four per day. The duration of therapy is dependent on the severity of the ulceration, but should not be for more than 8 weeks. It should be emphasised that this treatment reduces the severity but does not cure the condition which will continue to recur. There is no evidence that it causes serious sytemic effects, even in the elderly.

Moniliasis

An important manifestation of reduced salivary secretion and immunological impairment is oral moniliasis. The condition is even more prevalent where the elderly patient in hospital has diabetes, or where antibiotic therapy has allowed monilial overgrowth by destroying normal commensal organisms. Gentian violet was effective in this condition, but produced unsightly staining, particularly in old people who were muddled or who dribbled from the corner of a drooping mouth. It thus was supplanted by nystatin tablets. If these are used, it is important that the patient be instructed to allow them to dissolve in his mouth. Since nystatin is not absorbed it acts merely locally. Poor compliance on this may seriously impede the efficacy of the drug.

In a few patients moniliasis extends to involve the oesophagus. The condition is identified by a history of dysphagia and characteristic radiological changes. It also may respond to nystatin tablets. A recently prepared drug, the antifungal agent clotrimazole offers an alternative approach. It is useful in the treatment of systemic moniliasis, but its usefulness is limited by severe side-effects which include nausea, vomiting, and diarrhoea, hepatic impairment, and bone marrow suppression. Side-effects can be eliminated if the drug is given in a much lower dosage as a lozenge and the patient is asked to keep this in his mouth. With this, a dose of 50 mg five times daily is sufficient to eliminate oropharyngeal moniliasis. It remains to be seen whether age changes in renal and hepatic function may modify the good safety record which the lozenges have in younger patients.

Nutritional Glossitis and Stomatitis

Many old people have red, atrophic, and fissured tongues. Since many of them also suffer from iron, folic acid, or cyanocobalamin deficiency, clinicians assumed that in old age glossitis and nutrient deficiency were related. Most studies, however, have failed to establish that treatment with haematinics has any beneficial effect on tongue changes. This illustrates the danger in assuming a cause and effect relationship between two phenomena in old people with multiple pathology.

Another example is the concurrence of vitamin C deficiency and sublingual "petechiae" in old age. The tongue changes were at one time thought to result from ruptured capillaries in subclinical scurvy. Histological examination, however, has confirmed that the "petechiae" actually are dilated venules associated with ageing. Vitamin C deficiency and dilated venules then are only related to each other through the common variable of ageing.

A further clinical sign which now is not thought to be related to subnutrition is angular stomatitis, a condition in which the angles of the lips become soft and excoriated. Both angular stomatitis and riboflavine deficiency are common in old age, but bear no close relationship to each other.

Suppurative Parotitis

One of the most serious consequences of poor oral hygiene is suppurative parotitis. Improved standards of living and community health care have eliminated this problem in children and young or middle-aged adults, but it still occurs in old people, particularly if they are living alone and suffering from severe mental incapacity. Though the infection often is due to *Staphylococcus aureus* or *Streptococcus pyogenes,* Gram-negative organisms may be responsible, particularly if the patient has been on an antibiotic for a coincidental urinary or respiratory infection. Old people should be treated, therefore, with large doses of flucloxacillin and ampicillin (see Chap. 5).

Early identification of old people "at risk" is the best way of preventing them from neglecting oral hygiene, becoming dehydrated and thus developing a parotitis. Inappropriate medication also may contribute to the problem. Thus, a variety of drugs with an anticholinergic effect seriously impede salivary flow. They include bladder relaxants, tricyclic antidepressants, and phenothiazines or butyrophenone tranquillisers. Diuretics used with undue enthusiasm also may dry out the mouth.

Presbyoesophagus

A barium swallow in an elderly patient may demonstrate coincidental abnormal smooth muscle contractions. Oesophageal motility was investigated in detail in a group of nonagenarians suffering from a variety of conditions including mild dementia, diabetes, ischaemic heart disease, and anaemia. In them, normal peristaltic movements were impaired, and replaced by non-propulsive, often repetitive (tertiary) contractions (Soergel et al. 1964). The manometric pattern closely resembled that found in diffuse spasm of the oesophagus, a condition characterised by dysphagia and severe bouts of chest pain.

The question arises as to whether dysphagia, a common symptom in old age, might often be related to tertiary contractions, and whether this might respond to treatment with cholinergic drugs. The answer would appear to be in the negative, since most of the patients in the initial study were asymptomatic and the clinical experience of most doctors is that symptomatic diffuse spasm of the oesophagus is a rare entity in old age. Further, a more recent study in healthy old men failed to identify abnormal oesophageal motility patterns (Hollis and Castel 1974). This suggests that abnormal motility is related to diseases such as diabetes or dementia rather than ageing per se.

References

Connell AM, Hilton C, Irvine G, Lennard-Jones JE, Miesewicz IJ (1965) Variation in bowel habit in two population samples. Br Med J 2: 1095–1099

Davies DM (1977) Textbook of adverse drug reactions. Oxford University Press, Oxford, pp 156–159

Eastwood HDH (1971) Causes of jaundice in the elderly. Geront Clin 13: 69–81

Evans JG, Acheson ED (1965) An epidemiological study of ulcerative colitis and regional enteritis in the Oxford area. Gut 6: 311–324

Hollis J, Castell DO (1974) Oesophageal function in elderly men: a new look at presbyesophagus. Ann Int Med 80: 371–374

Kyle J (1971) An epidemiological study of Crohn's disease in North-East Scotland. Gastroenterology 61: 826–833

Lieber MM (1952) The incidence of gallstones and their correlation with other disease. Ann Surg 135: 394–399

MacGregor CGA, Ogg LJ, Smith IS, Cochran AJ, Gray GR, Gillespie G, Forrester J (1977) Immunological and other laboratory studies of patients receiving short-term cimetidine therapy. Lancet 1: 122–123

Montgomery RD, Haeney MR, Ross IN, Sammons HG, Basford AV, Balakishnan S, Mayer PP, Culank LS, Field J, Gesling P (1978) The ageing gut: a study of intestinal absorption in relation to the elderly. Q J Med 47: 197–211

Parks TG (1969) Natural history of diverticular disease of the colon. A review of 521 cases. Br Med J 4: 639–642

Pentland B, Pennington CR (1980) Acute diarrhoea in the elderly. Age Ageing 9: 90–92

Price HL, Gazzard BG, Dawson AM (1977) Steatorrhoea in the elderly. Br Med J 1: 1582–1584

Pridie RB (1966) Incidence and coincidence of hiatus hernia. Gut 7: 188–189

Richter JE, Castell DO (1981) Current approaches in the medical treatment of oesophageal reflux. Drugs 21: 283–291

Soergel KH, Zboralske FF, Amberg JR (1964) Presbyesophagus: esophageal motility in nonogerians. J Clin Invest 43: 1472–1479

Watkinson G (1960) The incidence of chronic peptic ulcer found at necrospsy. Gut 1: 14–20

7 Bladder Disorders

Physiology and Pharmacology of the Bladder

The main function of the bladder is to provide control over the storage and voiding of urine. Important elements of the system are the detrusor muscle, the trigone, the urethra, and the periurethral muscles (Fig. 7.1).

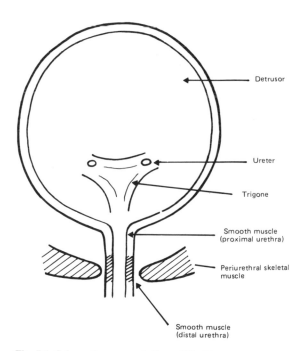

Detrusor

Ureter

Trigone

Smooth muscle
(proximal urethra)

Periurethral skeletal
muscle

Smooth muscle
(distal urethra)

Fig. 7.1. Schematic representation of bladder anatomy.

During the storage phase, the detrusor relaxes to accommodate increasing volumes of urine until the mechanical limits of distensibility are reached. Voiding, in turn, is the result of detrusor contraction.

The trigone forms the base of the bladder and is linked to both the ureters and the urethra. While the bladder is filling the trigone is flat, but during voiding it assumes a funnel shape with the urethra at the base of the funnel. This produces maximum levels of pressure in the urethra so that micturition is facilitated.

Relaxation and constriction of the urethra also plays an important part in bladder control. The proximal part of the urethra contains smooth muscle, which merges with skeletal muscle in the more distal part. Contraction of periurethral skeletal muscle also facilitates bladder control. Recent evidence suggests that the concept of internal and external urethral sphincters is no longer appropriate.

Parasympathetic nerves travel from the spinal cord to the pelvic ganglia where they synapse with postganglionic neurones (Fig. 7.2). These promote smooth muscle contractions in the detrusor and relaxation of both smooth and skeletal muscle in the urethra, and the neurotransmitter at both the ganglia and neuromuscular junctions is acetylcholine. At the latter site its action can be blocked by atropine.

The sympathetic nerves travel from the spinal cord to two chains of ganglia.

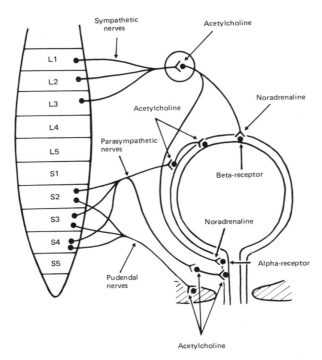

Fig. 7.2. Schematic representation of efferent innervation of the bladder.

Thence presynaptic fibres travel to alpha and beta catecholamine receptors in the detrusor and urethra. At the ganglia the neurotransmitter is acetylcholine, but here its action is not inhibited by atropine. Presynaptic fibres release noradrenaline which interacts with alpha-receptors to cause smooth muscle contractions and with beta-receptors to cause small muscle relaxation. Since most alpha-receptors are in the urethra and most beta-receptors in the detrusor, the effect of the sympathetic nervous system is to promote storage.

Motor nerves to skeletal muscle travel from the spinal cord through the pudendal nerve to the periurethral muscles. Here, acetylcholine released at the neuromuscular junction is not inactivated by atropine.

Afferent fibres from the bladder travel via both pudendal and parasympathetic nerves to the spinal cord, then up through the lateral spinothalamic tracts to the cerebral cortex, where they convey a sensation of either fullness or voiding. The way in which the cortex and hypothalamus regulates bladder function is unclear, but the predominant effect appears to be that of detrusor relaxation and urethral contraction.

Urinary Incontinence

The first stage in the treatment of urinary incontinence is to identify the cause (Table 7.1). In old age this frequently is due to damage in the cerebral cortex so that inhibitory impulses no longer travel to the sacral parasympathetic nervous system. In this situation, the bladder fails to relax as it fills, so that the intravesical pressure rises, and the patient has to void urine at a very low bladder volume. Damage to the spinal cord is a much less common cause for incontinence in the elderly. When this occurs there is complete loss of control and the bladder empties automatically at regular short intervals. If afferent or efferent impulses to or from the spinal cord are disturbed the bladder is large and atonic, dribbling urine continuously once its maximum volume has been reached. The classical cause of this was tabes dorsalis. Far more common causes in old people nowadays are diabetes mellitus and Parkinson's disease.

If there is clinical evidence to suggest that the patient has a neurogenic bladder, it is important to back this up by performing further investigations. The most useful is filling cystometrography. Accurate information on the intravesical pressure is collected by connecting a catheter from the bladder to a pressure transducer linked to a recorder. From this is subtracted the intra-abdominal pressure recorded from a catheter within the rectum. If this equipment is not available some idea of bladder function can be obtained by connecting a bladder catheter to a fluid reservoir and a water manometer. It will at least distinguish between an uninhibited bladder and an atonic one.

Local disturbances of the genito-urinary tract also are important causes of urinary incontinence. The urethra may be compressed by a faecal impaction or prostatic enlargement. Here a distended bladder produces an overflow incontinence.

Table 7.1. Causes of urinary incontinence in the elderly

Neurological abnormalities

Faulty cortical inhibition due to	a) Alzheimer's disease
	b) cerebrovascular disease
	c) frontal lobe tumour
	d) Parkinson's disease
Automatic bladder due to	a) meningioma of cord
	b) secondary tumour
	c) collapsed vertebral body
	d) spinal artery thrombosis
Atonic neuropathic bladder due to	a) diabetic autonomic neuropathy
	b) Parkinsonian neuropathy
	c) cauda equina lesion
	d) anticholinergic drugs
	e) tabes dorsalis

Polyuria

Diuretics

Local causes

Urinary retention due to	a) faecal impaction
	b) prostatic enlargement

Prolapse or cystocoele
Acute cystitis
Atrophic urethritis
Carcinoma of bladder
Bladder calculus

An acute urinary tract infection may cause frequency, urgency, and dysuria as well as urinary incontinence. This has to be distinguished from the asymptomatic bacteruria which inevitably occurs in disorders associated with incomplete emptying of the bladder. These often also cause urinary incontinence, but there is no direct association between the bacteruria and the incontinence.

Postmenopausal involutional changes in the vagina often are accompanied by similar changes in the urethra and trigone. These become atrophic, inflamed, and tender so that frequency, dysuria, and incontinence are common.

In the management of urinary incontinence, drug treatment is, at best, merely an adjunct to other forms of therapy. It is fundamental that an effective programme of education and toilet training be prescribed by the doctor and organised by the nursing staff. Practical procedures include clearance of faecal impaction, prostatectomy, pelvic floor repair, and irradiation of a bladder tumour.

Bladder Relaxants

One of the more important effects of the quaternary ammonium anticholinergic agents is that they increase bladder capacity and reduce the intravesical pressure. This has led to such drugs being widely used in the management of urinary incontinence related to an uninhibited bladder.

An example is that propantheline is used in a dose which usually starts at 15 mg three times daily, but may be gradually increased to a maximum of 45 mg three times daily. The pattern of the incontinence influences the timing of a dose. Thus, if a patient is wet at night, it is reasonable to give 30 mg at 8 p.m.

Like most quaternary ammonium salts, propantheline is poorly absorbed from the gut, being largely destroyed by first-pass metabolism through the liver. Despite its poor bio-availability, however, propantheline exerts potent pharmacological effects even when taken orally. The effects of ageing on absorption and pharmacological activity have not been studied yet.

Anticholinergic side-effects often prevent doctors from giving a dose optimal for maximum bladder relaxation (Table 7.2). In sick old people, a dry mouth associated with anticholinergic agents may lead to a nasty oral infection, sometimes going on to produce a suppurative parotitis. Meticulous oral hygiene, therefore, is at a premium in patients on these drugs.

Table 7.2. Side-effects of anticholinergic agents

Blurred vision
Dry mouth
Constipation
Urinary retention
Drowsiness
Glaucoma

Emepronium is another quaternary ammonium compound which has been used in urinary incontinence. A number of studies have provided evidence of its efficacy in both elderly men and women with incontinence (Brocklehurst et al. 1972). A later report produced evidence that while the drug had a potent effect on detrusor muscle when given parenterally, it had little effect when taken orally (Ritch et al. 1977). This was attributed to its poor gastro-intestinal absorption. Further investigation is required to resolve the debate.

The dosage recommended is 200 mg three times daily, but this often is increased to 400 mg in the hope that this will achieve maximal efficacy. The drug has most of the side-effects of propantheline, but an additional problem is that it has a local irritant effect. If an elderly patient is not cooperative the tablet may remain in his mouth and cause ulceration. Even if the tablet is swallowed, gastro-intestinal stasis may result in it causing oesophageal ulceration.

Flavoxate is a tertiary amine compound which is a potent smooth muscle relaxant. Its effect on the detrusor muscle is similar to that of propantheline, but it was weaker anticholinergic effects. Studies on incontinent patients suggested that its efficacy is comparable with that of emepronium (Stanton 1973). A subsequent study, however, found that in elderly patients neither intravenous nor oral flavoxate had an effect on urethral sphincter tone, bladder pressure at capacity, detrusor spasm, or the severity of incontinence (Briggs et al. 1980). As with emepronium, further study will be required to resolve the conflicting evidence. If flavoxate is used, it should be given orally in a dose of 200 mg three times daily.

An alternative approach is to make use of the alpha-adrenergic agonist and anticholinergic properties of an antidepressant. Imipramine, when used in incontinent elderly patients, has a pronounced effect on intravesical pressure, detrusor spasms, and urethral pressure. If further experience establishes its value in this field, it will probably be given in a single evening dose of between 50 and 100 mg, starting with an initial dose of 25 mg and increasing by 25-mg stages. The prolonged half-life of the drug ensures that in addition to effecting control of nocturnal incontinence it continues to reduce the intravesical pressure for most of the following day. The major disadvantage to this approach is that tricyclic antidepressants have many side-effects, so that they have to be withdrawn in a sizeable proportion of elderly patients.

A recently developed smooth muscle relaxant is flunasizine. It is a calcium antagonist which has little effect on myocardial activity. Though an effect on bladder capacity has not been confirmed yet, there is evidence that it reduces both urgency and urinary incontinence in elderly women. An advantage over many other agents is that it has a long duration of action, so that it only has to be given once daily. The dosage suggested is 20 mg. Since the drug has a mild sedative effect it is best given in the evening. Further study is required to confirm its efficacy, and investigate it for possible side-effects such as peripheral oedema.

A variety of prostaglandins produce contraction of human bladder muscle in vitro. There is a theoretical basis, thus, for using a prostaglandin inhibitor in patients with an uninhibited bladder. Indomethacin has been used in this situation, but in doses adequate to inhibit prostaglandin synthesis it usually causes headaches and nausea.

The more recently developed non-steroidal anti-inflammatory agent flurbiprofen has the advantages over indomethacin of having a much lower toxicity and a much more potent inhibitory effect on prostaglandin synthesis. Given in a dose of 50 mg three times daily to women with detrusor instability flurbiprofen reduced both diurnal and nocturnal frequency, as well as improving urgency and urge incontinence. Though this represents a promising approach, further experience is required before it can be recommended for routine management in the neurogenic bladder.

In treating patients with an uninhibited bladder most attention has been given to reducing detrusor tone. Considerable benefit, however, might also be conferred by increasing the tone of the internal bladder sphincter. Alpha-sympatheticomimetic agents have this effect. One of these, ephedrine, has an effect comparable to that of propantheline. At present it is not widely used in the management of incontinence, but the time may have come for a reappraisal of its efficacy.

The present situation in the drug treatment of the uninhibited bladder in old age, then, is that for a long time, anticholinergic drugs have been the drugs of first choice in the management of the disorder. Recent studies on bladder function have challenged their right to this position, but further work is required before recommending that an alternative approach might be sought. Perhaps the most promising rivals to the anticholinergic agents are the tricyclic antidepressants and calcium antagonists, but their places remain to be established. Inhibitors of prostaglandin synthesis open up an exciting new field, but the drugs currently available have too high a level of side-effects, at the dosage required, for them to be of much practical value.

Agents Increasing Bladder Tone

Patients with incontinence resulting from loss of detrusor tone are best treated with drugs which cause smooth muscle contraction. One of these is bethanechol, a potent cholinergic agent which stimulates acetylcholine receptors in smooth muscle (Westmore 1979). If given to a patient with an atonic bladder it reduces the bladder volume and increases the intravesical pressure. Sometimes this allows the patient to initiate normal micturition again. At other times it merely converts a dribbling incontinence to frequent episodes of uncontrolled bladder emptying. The response to therapy depends upon whether or not the parasympathetic efferent/afferent reflex arc is incompletely or completely destroyed. The normal dose is 5 mg orally four times daily.

Bethanechol should not be used if there is evidence of an outflow obstruction. It stimulates postganglionic sympathetic nerve fibres supplying the urethra. Susceptible patients, thus, may develop an acute retention, associated with severe cramping pains due to detrusor spasm.

An alternative is to reduce outflow resistance using an adrenoceptor blocking agent. The decrease in urethral tone allows the bladder to empty more readily. Again, whether this achieves continence or merely modifies the pattern of incontinence depends upon the integrity of the autonomic nervous system.

The drug usually used is phenoxybenzamine in a dose of 5–10 mg three times daily. Unfortunately, it often causes postural hypotension and thus is tolerated poorly by old people.

There have been few reports on trials of drug treatment for an atonic bladder. This probably is because the condition is less common than the uninhibited bladder. It does, however, mean that statements on the efficacy of bethanechol or phenoxybenzamine are based on clinical impression rather than hard scientific evidence.

Hormones

If a patient has signs of atrophic vaginitis it is likely that her urethra and trigone also are involved. Her incontinence may be improved by the administration of oestrogens. Treatment may be given topically as 0.1% dienoestrol cream applied by an applicator twice daily for periods of up to 2 weeks. The advantage of local application is that this does not give rise to vaginal haemorrhage. Its disadvantage is that frail elderly women experience difficulty in using the applicator.

One of the most widely used oral oestrogens is ethinyloestradiol given in a dose of 10–20 μg daily. In the management of incontinence another hormone, quinestradol, may have advantages over ethinyloestradiol in that it reverses involutional changes in the genito-urinary tract without causing vaginal bleeding or systemic disturbances. If full benefit is to be obtained from the drug, its use should be limited to patients with clinical evidence of atrophic vaginitis. Indiscriminate use in all women with incontinence will give poor results. The dose is 500 μg twice daily for 6 weeks.

Antibiotics

Old people with an acute cystitis are likely to have symptoms of frequency, dysuria, and incontinence and their incontinence is likely to respond to an antibiotic. Most patients with urinary incontinence, however, have a bacteriuria which is related to the cause of the incontinence, e.g. incomplete emptying of an uninhibited bladder. Since antibiotics, in this situation, do not control the underlying cause, they cannot be expected to have any effect on the incontinence. They merely select out increasingly resistant organisms, which present dangers to both the patient and other people in the ward.

References

Briggs RS, Castleden CM, Asher MJ (1980) The effect of flavoxate on uninhibited detrusor contractions and urinary incontinence in the elderly. J Urol 123: 665–666
Brocklehurst JC, Armitage P, Johart AJ (1972) Emepronium bromide in urinary incontinence. Age Ageing 1: 152–157
Ritch AES, Castleden CM, George CF, Hall MRP (1977) A second look at emepronium bromide in urinary incontinence. Lancet 1: 504–506
Stanton S (1973) A comparison of emepronium bromide and flavoxate hydrochloride in the treatment of urinary incontinence. J Urol 110: 529–532
Westmore DD (1979) Urinary incontinence: which drugs to use. Drugs 17: 418–422

8 The Locomotor System

Bone Disorders

Osteoporosis

Ageing almost invariably is accompanied by a reduction in skeletal mass. In women this declines rapidly betwen the ages of 45 and 75 years, whereas in men the decline begins about 10 years later and then is far less steep. Clinical consequences are a high incidence of fractures of the lower end of the forearm in middle aged women, followed by an exponentially increasing incidence of fractured proximal femurs in elderly men and women (Fig. 8.1). Osteoporosis also results in the pain and deformity due to crush fractures of vertebral bodies. The simple treatment of bone loss is to use calcium supplements. These increase serum calcium concentrations and thus suppress secretion of parathyroid hormone and reduce levels of 1,25-dihydroxycholecalciferol (1,25 $[OH]_2D$), the renal metabolite of vitamin D. Follow-up studies have shown that this is effective in reducing the rate of bone resorption. The appropriate dose of a calcium salt is 1–1.5 g of elemental calcium daily. The theoretical risk here is that of producing renal calculi.

An important cause of bone loss in postmenopausal women is a decline in oestrogen concentrations. In the absence of oestrogens bone becomes increasingly sensitive to the effects of parathyroid hormone and 1,25 $[OH]_2D$. Calcium is resorbed from the skeleton and lost in the urine. In this situation treatment with oestrogens halts further bone loss. The agents in current use are listed in Table 8.1. These are taken for 21 days out of each 28-day cycle. The arrest of bone loss by oestrogens is followed by a reduced incidence of fractures of the distal end of the radius and proximal end of the femur. Against benefits of long-term oestrogen therapy some theoretical risks must be balanced. High doses may cause hypertension, stroke, myocardial infarction, hypertriglyceridaemia, sodium retention, and endometrial cancer. Large epidemiological studies are required to establish the relative advantages and disadvantages of this regime. One solution would be to limit the use of oestrogens to postmeno-

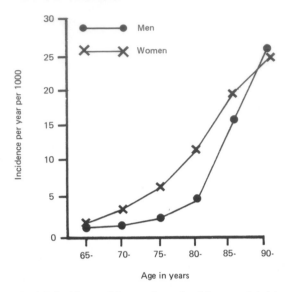

Fig. 8.1. Incidence of fractured proximal femurs related to age in Newcastle upon Tyne (Grimley Evans 1979).

pausal women with a high ratio of hydroxypraline to creatinine, indicative of an increased rate of skeletal demineralisation. It would be difficult, however, to use such a test routinely in all postmenopausal women.

A variety of anabolic steroids also have been used in the treatment of osteoporosis. In some trials they have been found to control symptoms such as the pain of crush fractures. A recent investigation produced evidence that, when given with calcium, the anabolic agent stanazolol may actually replace bone loss.

Though treatment with oestrogens, anabolic steroids, or calcium may be useful, other agents may be indicated in patients who exhibit clinical manifestations of osteoporosis. A popular approach in the USA is to make use of fluoride salts (Jowsey 1977). These increase the thickness of bone trabeculae by stimulating osteoblastic activity.

Table 8.1. Oestrogens used in the treatment of postmenopausal osteoporosis

Conjugated oestrogens	0.625 mg daily
Oestradiol valerate	2 mg daily
Ethinyloestradiol	15 μg daily
Piperazine oestrone sulphate	3 mg daily
Menophase pack	Tablets taken in sequence

Unfortunately, bone formed in this way is poorly calcified, so that osteoporosis may be corrected, but is replaced with osteomalacia. A solution to this is to add calcium to the medication. At one time the regime was supplemented further with large doses of vitamin D, but all that is done now is to give sufficient ergocalciferol to ensure that the intake of the vitamin is at the recommended norm for adults. The treatment in current use then is 62–88 mg sodium fluoride daily; 1.3 g elemental calcium daily; and 400 i.u. ergocalciferol daily. Continuing follow-up is necessary to establish whether increasing bone thickness in this way will reduce the incidence of fractures.

Many patients with osteoporosis have reduced plasma concentrations of 1,25[OH]$_2$D. A cause of this might be inpaired synthesis of the metabolite by ageing kidneys. Possible consequences would be a suboptimal absorption of calcium from the gut, resulting in there being insufficient calcium available for bone formation. Since the deficiency of calcium is marginal, this would give rise to osteoporosis (bone rarefaction) rather than skeletal decalcification (osteomalacia).

This has led to 1,25[OH]$_2$D (calcitriol) and the synthetic analogue 1α-hydroxycholecalciferol (1αOHD; alfacalcidol) being used in the treatment of osteoporosis. The clinical response has been disappointing owing to the hormones increasing resorption of calcium from bones as well as its absorption from the gut. A solution is to give alfacalcidol or calcitriol along with oestrogens. Here, however, serum calcium concentrations should be monitored to ensure that hypercalcaemia does not occur.

Despite the considerable amount of work on the treatment of osteoporosis performed over the last 10 years, comparatively little has emerged which is of direct value to the clinician. Oestrogen therapy seems to be of value in preventing osteoporosis, but the long-term risks have not been fully evaluated. Calcium supplements also may be useful but further work is required to establish their efficacy. At present they should only be given to patients with severe pain associated with crush fractures. Long-term evaluation of their role in preventing fractures of the radius and femur is required, before they can be recommended in the routine treatment of asymptomatic bone rarefaction.

Osteomalacia

A poor diet and low sunlight exposure lead to a high prevalence of vitamin D deficiency in elderly women. Florid cases present with bone pain, muscle weakness, low serum calcium and phosphate and high serum alkaline phosphatase concentrations and radiological evidence of Looser's zones. This can be treated effectively by giving a single intramuscular injection of 600 000 units (2 ml) of calciferol. An alternative is to give calciferol solution orally in a dose of 3000 units daily. The disadvantage of this approach is that frail elderly patients have poor compliance.

It is important that patients on large oral doses of vitamin D be kept under regular review and serum calcium concentrations checked regularly. The effects of calciferol-induced hypercalcaemia include confusion, anorexia, vomiting, diarrhoea, renal calculi, and renal failure. Alfacalcidol and calcitriol are also effective in osteomalacia, but in the absence of renal impairment have no advantage over the parent substance.

Many old people have low serum concentrations of 25-hydroxycholecalciferol (25OHD) despite the fact that their serum concentrations of calcium, phosphate, and alkaline phosphatase are normal. Again many patients with fractured proximal femurs who have normal serum calcium, phosphate, and alkaline phosphatase concentrations have histological evidence of skeletal decalcification. The question arises as to whether such individuals with early vitamin D deficiency should be given supplements. It is logical to suppose that if patients with low serum 25OHD concentrations were followed for long enough they would eventually develop clinical signs of the deficiency. Though positive evidence of this is not available yet, a case could be made for giving vitamin D to elderly patients who were housebound. This could be given as one tablet of calcium and vitamin D (500 units of calciferol) BPC daily. Plasma 25OHD concentrations may also be elevated by exposing patients to an artificial ultraviolet light source. This has been used with variable success in long-stay hospitals, but is not of much practical value in individual houses.

Paget's Disease

Paget's disease is common in the elderly and often presents incidentally as a radiological abnormality or an elevated serum alkaline phosphatase concentration. Effective forms of treatment are now available but since these are expensive and involve careful monitoring they should only be given to patients with symptoms (Table 8.2). It also is important that, in an individual patient, the symptom and Paget's disease are not merely coincidental. There is no point in treating presbycousis with calcitonin, or cardiac failure due to mitral incompetence with diphosphonates.

Table 8.2. Complications of Paget's disease

Bone pain
Bone deformity
Bone fracture
Osteogenic sarcoma
Deafness
Midbrain and cord compression
High output cardiac failure

Calcitonin

Calcitonin is a hormone produced by the parafollicular cells of the thyroid gland. The most important clinical effect is that it inhibits osteoclastic activity, and thus reduces bone turnover. This is of importance in Paget's disease where there is an increase of both osteoclastic and osteoblastic activity. The hormone, when given parenterally for several months, reduces bone turnover, so that the coarse unstructured architecture of affected bone is completely remodelled, and a normal radiological pattern restored. Diminished bone turnover also is reflected by the restoration of high serum alkaline phosphatase concentrations to normal. This index thus provides a useful means of monitoring a response to treatment.

Complications of Paget's disease in which calcitonin is particularly useful are bone pain, fractures, and neurological compressed syndromes. Deafness, unfortunately, often does not respond to treatment. The agent also is useful if given along with surgery to correct major bone and joint deformities.

Both calcitonin, from a porcine source, and salcatonin, from a salmon one, are available for routine use. Dosage is dependent upon the severity of symptoms, but a reasonable approach would be to give 100 units subcutaneously daily until symptomatic and biochemical remission is achieved, and then reduce this to 100 units twice or three times weekly. Salcatonin is less likely to stimulate antibody formation than porcine calcitonin and thus can usually be given at less frequent intervals. Treatment is continued for 6 months. When this is stopped, the alkaline phosphatase rises again, but the drug should only be reintroduced if there is clinical deterioration. Antibodies sometimes suppress calcitonin activity and if this happens the use of human calcitonin should be considered.

Side-effects of calcitonin include malaise, flushing urticaria, sneezing, nausea, vomiting, and diarrhoea. Subcutaneous injections are less likely to cause these than intramuscular ones.

Diphosphonate

A diphosphonate is a substance which, after absorption from the gut, forms a film over exposed surfaces of bone, where it inhibits the formation and dissolution of hydroxyapatite crystals. In Paget's disease, it reduces bone turnover and is effective in restoring the bone architecture to normal and depressing the serum alkaline phosphatase concentration. Unfortunately, bone mineralisation also is inhibited and patients on treatment may develop histological signs of osteomalacia. This can be tackled by reducing the dose of diphosphonate, but the therapeutic index between reduced bone turnover and reduced mineralisation is narrow, so that it is difficult to use the drug in routine clinical practice.

Two compounds related to diphosphonate which suppress bone turnover without altering mineralisation have now been developed. These are (3-amino-1-hydroxypropylidene)-1,1-diphosphonate (ADP) and dichloromethylene diphosphonate (Cl_2MDP). Both are effective in the treatment of Paget's disease when taken orally. The dose of ADP is $30\,\mu mol/kg$ body weight for 30 days followed by a maintenance dose of $15\,\mu mol/kg$. This has occasionally to be increased to $30\,\mu mol/kg$ to maintain remission. With Cl_2MDP, effective remission is achieved by giving 1600 mg/day.

Further research is required to assess the relative roles of calcitonin and diphosphonates in Paget's disease, the place for combination therapy, and any differences in the response of old people to diphosphonates.

Mithramycin

This antimitotic antibiotic is effective in suppressing osteoblastic and osteoclastic activity. It may therefore be used in treating Paget's disease. Its serious effects in the bone marrow and on renal and hepatic function mean that it should rarely, if ever, be used for this purpose in the elderly.

Drugs Causing Bone Disorders

Corticosteroids

Corticosteroids reduce bone mass by inhibiting osteoblastic activity and reducing the intestinal absorption of calcium. The likelihood of such bone loss causing problems relates to the bone mass present at the start of treatment. Thus old people and, in particular, old women are at particular risk. The duration of steroid therapy also is important and is the explanation for the prohibitively high incidence of fractures in elderly women on prolonged steroid treatment. The simplest answer to the problem is to think carefully before giving steroids to old people. If corticosteroids have to be given, consideration should be given to improving calcium absorption by using either alfacalcidol or calcitriol. Serum calcium concentrations then have to be monitored closely.

Anticonvulsants

Phenytoin and phenobarbitone may cause osteomalacia by increasing the hepatic metabolism of vitamin D. The problem originally was highlighted in epileptic children but, obviously, housebound elderly people are also at risk. It is reasonable, therefore, to give frail old people on anticonvulsants calciferol supplements, say, 500 units of calciferol daily (as calcium with vitamin D tablets BPC).

Joint Disorders

Rheumatoid Arthritis

Though rheumatoid arthritis has a peak incidence in youth and early middle age, its long-term effects frequently persist into old age. These include secondary osteoarthritis, joint subluxation or disorganisation, hand and foot deformities, bone rarefaction, muscle wasting, and systemic changes such as pulmonary fibrosis, polyneuropathy, and subnutrition.

In about 10% of cases, rheumatoid arthritis develops for the first time in patients of 60 years and over. Usually the symptoms and signs are similar to those found in younger patients, but a quarter of subjects present with features characteristic of the syndrome of "benign rheumatoid arthritis of the aged" (Corrigan et al. 1974). Here the condition is heralded by a severe polyarthralgia associated with constitutional disorders such as anorexia, weight loss, malaise, and depression. The erythrocyte sedimentation rate is markedly elevated, while the haemoglobin, serum albumin, serum iron, and serum total iron binding capacity often are low. Limb girdle pain and stiffness similar to that found in polymyalgia rheumatica may be prominent. High titres for rheumatoid factor are the rule. The prognosis is excellent and most patients are in complete remission by 18 months.

Drug treatment of rheumatoid arthritis depends upon its presentation. If the condition is long-standing, pain and disability may be due to joint deformity rather than active disease. Evidence of this should be sought by testing for joint tenderness and soft tissue swelling and by measuring the erythrocyte sedimentation rate or the level of C-reactive protein. Only if these are abnormal should agents such as gold, corticosteroids, or powerful anti-inflammatory analgesics be considered. Pain due to deformity or osteoarthritis should respond to paracetamol or to small doses of less potent anti-inflammatory analgesics.

If there is evidence of synovial inflammation, drugs used in younger patients should be considered also in the elderly, but particular attention should be given to the problems of poor compliance, increased toxicity, and interactions with other preparations.

The drugs of first choice in an exacerbation of rheumatoid arthritis are the non-steroidal anti-inflammatory agents. They probably act by inhibiting prostaglandin synthesis. In doing this they also interfere with the ability of prostacyclin to increase gastric mucosal blood flow and reduce acid secretion, thus increasing the risk of mucosal erosion and ulceration. Gastric irritation thus is a necessary concomitant in the activity of most anti-inflammatory agents, and can never be eliminated completely. Despite this some agents are more irritant than others. This has led to the development of a bewildering host of non-steroidal anti-inflammatory agents.

Aspirin

This is the standard non-steroidal agent against which all others are compared. It causes a very high incidence of dyspepsia and gastric erosions and ulcers. The risk is increased in ascorbic acid deficiency, so that if an elderly person has to be on regular doses of aspirin it is important to supplement his diet. Gastric irritation also may be reduced by using soluble or enteric-coated aspirin, or a more complex compound such as benorylate (a salicylate-paracetamol ester) or choline magnesium trisalicylate (a trisalicylate compound activated by metabolism into three salicylate radicals in the liver). These preparations do not eliminate the systemic side-effects of salicylates. In old people the most important of these is ototoxicity associated with ataxia and deafness (Ballantyne 1970).

Pyrazoles

Phenylbutazone and oxyphenbutazone are potent anti-inflammatory agents, but their side-effects are of such severity that they should not be used in the long-term treatment of rheumatoid arthritis in the elderly. An uncommon but worrying complication is an irreversible and fatal aplastic anaemia (Fig. 8.2). The pyrazoles also often cause gastric erosions and ulcers associated with anaemia and haematemesis, whilst their effect on fluid retention makes them particularly dangerous in old people with cardiac disease. Since they have a high affinity for albumin, they can cause dangerous interactions in patients on other protein-bound drugs. Examples of these include the coumarin anticoagulants and sulphonurea hypoglycaemic agents.

More recently developed pyrazoles include feprazone and azapropazone. These are effective as anti-inflammatory agents, but have most of the side-effects of phenylbutazone. An exception is that they do not cause aplastic anaemia.

Indoles and Related Compounds

Indomethacin is another potent anti-inflammatory agent. The high incidence of gastro-intestinal disturbance, ulceration, blood loss, and fluid retention means

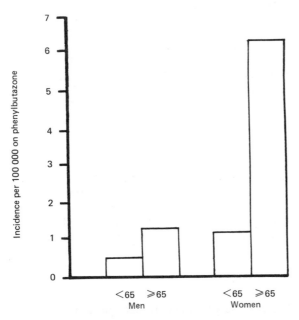

Fig. 8.2. Death rate from aplastic anaemia due to phenylbutazone related to age and sex (Inman 1977).

that it should not normally be used as a drug of first choice in the treatment of rheumatoid arthritis in the elderly. A particular problem in old people is that it often causes neurological disturbances, which include headache, drowsiness, and mental confusion. Despite its affinity for albumin, indomethacin is comparatively rarely involved in drug interactions.

Sulindac has a particularly long duration of action, in that though it itself has a half-life of only 8 h it is metabolised into an active sulphide with half-life of 16 h. This is useful in old people since it need only be given twice a day. The drug can cause gastro-intestinal blood loss and dyspepsia, but these are much less frequent or severe than those with aspirin, phenylbutazone or indomethacin. It sometimes also causes headache or drowsiness, but these symptoms are mild and rarely warrant discontinuation of therapy. The dosage is 100–200 mg twice daily.

Tolmetin, another related compound, has relatively few side-effects, but its relatively short half-life means that it has no particular advantage over the wide range of other anti-inflammatory agents currently available.

Propionic Acid Derivatives

These drugs also cause many fewer gastro-intestinal side-effects and blood loss than aspirin, phenylbutazone, or indomethacin, and are effective analgesic and anti-inflammatory agents. They include naproxen, ibuprofen, fenoprofen, ketoprofen, flurbiprofen, and fenbrufen. In old age, naproxen and fenbrufen have a marginal advantage over the others in that they have longer half-lives and thus can be given twice rather than three times daily.

Diclofenac, Fenclofenac, and Piroxicam

The efficacy and range of side-effects for these drugs is similar to that of the propionic acid derivatives. Fenclofenac has a half-life of 12–21 h, and piroxicam has one of up to 36–48 h. They thus need only be given twice daily and are particularly useful in the elderly.

Fenamates

Mefenamic and flufenamic acid often cause gastro-intestinal disturbances and, in particular, diarrhoea. In old people this can lead to serious dehydration. This combined with a direct toxic effect on the renal medulla may lead to a nephropathy manifesting itself as a rising blood urea and reduced urinary concentrating ability. They thus should not be used in the routine treatment of rheumatoid arthritis in old age.

Selection of Anti-inflammatory Agents

If the clinician is to make effective use of non-steroidal anti-inflammatory agents in rheumatoid arthritis, he must adhere to several general principles. The first is to start with a drug with a low toxicity. Examples include the propionic acid derivatives, and diclofenac, fenclofenac, and piroxicam. He may then decide to use an agent which can be given twice rather than three times daily and concentrate therefore on naproxen, fenbrufen, fenclofenac and prioxicam. Only one drug should be used at a time and normally it takes 2–3 weeks for it to become fully effective. Quite apart from the fact that multiple analgesic therapy shows no advantage in rheumatoid arthritis, old people have the ubiquitous problem of polypharmacy.

If, after 3 weeks, the drug has not relieved symptoms, it should be changed for another agent. Patients show a wide and variable response to different anti-inflammatory agents, so that although one does not work another may well be effective. There is no cross-sensitivity between the propionic acid derivatives so that, if desired, several of these may be tried in succession. Normally up to four agents should be tried before deciding that the milder non-steroidal agents are ineffective. It then may be necessary to give either aspirin or indomethacin.

Second-Line Drugs

If none of the non-steroidal agents produces effective control, consideration should be given to using second-line agents. These often take several weeks to achieve an effect, and most have a high level of toxicity. They should only be used in old people if they are likely to (1) relieve pain not controlled by other means, (2) produce a significant improvement in the self-care capacity, or (3) control severe systemic effects. Elderly patients with long-standing "burnt out" rheumatoid arthritis rarely require them, those with typical rheumatoid arthritis of recent onset sometimes require them, and those with severe benign rheumatoid arthritis of the aged often require them.

Gold. Salts of gold have been investigated extensively in the treatment of rheumatoid arthritis. They relieve clinical symptoms and signs in a large proportion of cases. In addition they slow the rate at which bone and articular surfaces are destroyed. Their major drawback is a high rate of side-effects (Table 8.3). Those causing most problems are skin rashes, marrow depression, and renal damage. Skin rashes usually resolve within 3 months of stopping treatment. Leucopenia and thrombocytopenia also usually resolve, but aplastic anaemia can be unremittant and fatal. Renal glomerular damage usually can be reversed by stopping treatment.

The question arises as to whether these problems are more likely to occur in the elderly. No information is available on whether the pharmacokinetics of gold salts are affected by ageing. Again it is uncertain whether age-related changes in renal function increase the risks of nephrotoxicity. All that can be said is that the side-effects of chrysotherapy are predictable and can be carefully monitored. From this point of view gold salts have an advantage over many other second-line therapies when treating rheumatoid arthritis in the elderly.

The standard preparation is sodium aurothiomalate given intramuscularly in weekly doses of 50 mg for 20 weeks. These then are progressively reduced to once every 4 weeks. Toxicity should be monitored before each injection by

Table 8.3. Side-effects of chrysotherapy

Side-effect	Incidence
Skin reactions (urticaria, lichen planus, pityriasis rosea, erythema nodosum, exfoliative dermatitis)	50%
Stomatitis	Common
Arthralgia and myalgia	15%
Leucopenia	1%
Aplastic anaemia	Rare
Thrombocytopenia	Uncommon
Proteinuria (membranous glomerulopathy)	2%–10%
Cholestatic jaundice	Rare
Enterocolitis	Uncommon
Pulmonary fibrosis	Rare
Corneal ulceration	Rare
Gold deposits in cornea	75%

looking at the skin and mouth, checking the full blood count including platelets, and checking for protein in the urine.

Corticosteroids. In the elderly, corticosteroid therapy should be limited to patients in whom non-steroidal anti-inflammatory drugs and gold have failed to achieve effective relief. Even then the possible benefits of treatment have to be balanced against the probable risks of side-effects. These are listed in Table 8.4.

Table 8.4. Side-effects of corticosteroid therapy

Proximal myopathy	Insomnia
Osteoporosis	Anxiety
Activation of diabetes	Mood changes
Hypertension	Confusion
Congestive cardiac failure	Reactivation of infection
Peptic ulceration	Breakdown of wounds and pressure areas

Since old people with rheumatoid arthritis may already be suffering from muscle weakness, bone rarefaction, hypertension, cardiac disease, carbohydrate intolerance, depression, mental impairment, quiescent tuberculosis, and a friable ischaemic skin, they obviously run a particularly high risk of running into trouble when on corticosteroid therapy. If the patient is suffering from multiple pathology, corticosteroids may interact with several of the other drugs which he is taking (Table 8.5).

Table 8.5. Drugs interacting with corticosteroids

Drug	Effect
Ephedrine	Increased corticosteroid clearance
Rifampicin	Increased corticosteroid clearance
Salicylates	Increased metabolism of salicylates
Insulin and oral hypoglycaemic drugs	Decreased glucose tolerance
Diuretics	Hypokalaemia

If corticosteroids have to be used in rheumatoid arthritis they should be started in small doses, say, 2.5 mg prednisolone daily, gradually increasing this until effective control of symptoms is achieved. Once the condition has been stabilised, an attempt should be made to withdraw therapy. Since this is likely to cause reactivation of symptoms, withdrawal should be very gradual say, 1 mg daily of prednisolone every month. Corticosteroids sometimes are given on alternate days. This has the theoretical advantage of allowing pituitary-adrenal activation at intervals between dosage. It complicates medication, however, and may lead to errors in the elderly.

Other Second-Line Treatments.   Many other drugs may be used in the long-term treatment of rheumatoid arthritis, but since most have serious side-effects it is difficult to justify their use on old people with multiple pathology and a limited life expectancy. Penicillamine can cause severe skin rashes, a 10% incidence of proteinuria and a 5% one of thrombocytopenia. Chloroquine causes severe retinopathy in 15% of patients. Side-effects from levamisole occur in 40% of treated subjects and include skin rashes, a flu-like illness, gastro-intestinal upsets, and agranulocytosis. Lastly, there are cytotoxic agents such as azathioprine, cyclophosphamide, and methotrexate. Their unpleasant side-effects include gastro-intestinal upsets, activation of infections, and bone marrow complications.

Osteoarthritis

Loss of articular cartilage, eburnation of opposing bone surfaces, and osteo-phyte formation at joint margins are so common in the elderly that it is probable that they form part of the ageing process. The correlation between clinical signs and symptoms and radiological changes often is poor. Thus a knee joint which is tender to touch and has grossly limited flexion and extension may have only minimal radiological evidence of loss of articular cartilage. It is likely that some factor additional to degeneration is responsible for the clinical picture. A possibility is that disintegrating cartilage releases irritant crystals of hydroxyapatite into the synovial fluid and that these set up an intense inflammatory response.

This would explain why even mild non-steroidal anti-inflammatory drugs are more effective than simple analgesics in the treatment of osteoarthritis.

The approach to drug treatment in osteoarthritis is similar to that for rheumatoid arthritis. One of the newer anti-inflammatory agents with low gastro-intestinal side-effects should be tried and switched for another one if it is ineffective. If none of these work it is doubtful whether recourse should be made to more powerful agents such as aspirin, phenylbutazone, or indomethacin. Quite apart from their high toxicity, there is a danger that by their very effectiveness they may allow too much use to be made of a joint. This may result in disorganisation of the joint and, if the hip joint is involved, avascular necrosis of the femoral head. For similar reasons both systemic and intra-articular corticosteroids should not be used in osteoarthritis.

Drug treatment has no effect on the underlying degenerative process in osteoarthritis, and hip and knee joint replacement increasingly is seen as an option, even in the very old.

Gout

The management of an acute exacerbation of gout in old age is similar to that for any age (Scott 1977). Indomethacin can be given as 50 mg four times daily. Since such high doses need only be given for several days, serious toxic effects are unlikely.

Once the acute attack has settled, it is wise merely to observe the patient rather than start long-term allopurinol or uricosuric agents. The limited life expectancy of old people is such that they may well die from unrelated disorders before they have another attack. Allopurinol and uricosuric agents should be avoided also in patients with asymptomatic hyperuricaemia. Old people often have a high serum uric acid concentration, particularly if they are on a diuretic, but this rarely causes trouble.

Muscular Disorders

Fibrositis

Many old people suffer from aches and pains in their neck, shoulders, and back. This may be associated with tender nodules overlying muscles, but physical and, indeed, laboratory and radiological examination is otherwise negative. The pathogenesis of the condition is unknown, but psychosocial factors such as anxiety, loneliness, and even depression may be important.

Drugs should be chosen with extreme care. Patients with such symptoms run the risk of becoming habituated to sedatives or tranquillisers and, more immediately, suffer from drowsiness and ataxia. Again, anti-inflammatory agents are unlikely to have any benefit over simple analgesics and are more likely to cause side-effects.

Amongst the simple analgesics, paracetamol is the drug of choice. Drugs such as dextropropoxyphene, though more potent, tend to be addictive. Sudden withdrawal, particularly in the elderly, may result in alarming psychotic disturbances.

Collagen Disorders

Sanctions against the use of corticosteroids in the elderly do not apply to patients with connective tissue diseases such as disseminated lupus erythematosus or polyarteritis nodosa. They are suffering from life-threatening disorders which should be treated promptly with corticosteroids and, where appropriate, with immunosuppressant drugs.

Polymyalgia Rheumatica

This is an inflammatory condition involving the muscles of the shoulder and pelvic girdles. It is closely related to giant cell arteritis, so that between 6% and 50% of patients with polymyalgia rheumatica have positive temporal artery biopsies. Thus, correct identification and treatment of the disorder results not only in controlling a painful and disabling disorder—it also prevents devastating complications of temporal arteritis such as retinal artery thrombosis or a cerebrovascular accident.

Both conditions respond promptly and effectively to corticosteroids, but until recently there was debate about the correct dosage. All authorities agreed that temporal arteritis should be treated with doses of prednisone between 45 and 60 mg/day, but some felt that patients presenting with polymyalgia rheumatica alone only required between 10 and 15 mg/day. Others felt that, since many of these patients had underlying arteritis, all should be given large doses of corticosteroids. Opinions about the length of treatment also were divided, ranging between 6 months and 5 years.

Jones and Hazleman (1981) found that the incidence of arteritic complications was extremely high in polymyalgia and that these occurred even if a temporal artery biopsy was negative. They recommended, therefore, that all patients be treated with between 45 and 60 mg of prednisone daily. They warned, however, that such a large dose would produce complications in the elderly.

The starting does of prednisone, then, should be between 45 and 60 mg/day, but if after 4 weeks there is a remission the dose should be reduced slowly to a maintenance one of 10 mg/day. If clinical signs relapse or the erythrocyte sedimentation rate rises the dose should be increased. After 1 year, if the condition remains under control, an attempt should be made to withdraw corticosteroids. Esselinckx et al. (1977) found no evidence that gradual withdrawal reduced the risk of relapse. They suggested therefore that treatment be stopped abruptly. Once this has been done the patient should be followed up with clinical and laboratory assessment for at least a year to ensure that there is no recurrence.

Metabolic and Drug-Induced Myopathies

Drugs are responsible for a wide range of muscular abnormalities (Table 8.6). Fortunately, most of these are rare and, in the elderly, the most common cause is hypokalaemia. This usually is related to diuretic therapy, but occasionally it is encountered in laxative abuse. Carbenoxolone has a mineralocorticoid effect and therefore should not be used in old people (Chap. 6). Other drugs commonly causing a myopathy are the corticosteroids. This is yet another reason for avoiding these in the elderly.

A wide range of drugs may block neuromuscular transmission but are only likely to cause serious problems in patients with a predisposition to myasthenia gravis.

Inborn errors of metabolism give rise to a wide range of myopathies. It would be interesting to investigate whether enzyme deficiencies due to ageing and disease produce similar disorders. At present the only metabolic disorder commonly causing a proximal myopathy is vitamin D deficiency. Patients suffering from this have weakness in their thigh muscles. This makes it difficult for them to rise from a chair and gives them a characteristic waddling gait. Administration of vitamin D usually produces a dramatic improvement in the performance of the patient.

Table 8.6. Drug-induced muscle syndromes

Disorder	Drugs implicated
Acute/subacute painful proximal myopathy	Drugs causing hypokalaemia: diuretics, purgatives, carbenoxolone Cimetidine Bumetanide
Subacute/chronic painless proximal myopathy	Corticosteroids Drugs causing hypokalaemia: see above
Myasthenic syndrome	Aminoglycosides Tetracyclics Propranolol Phenytoin Chlorpromazine Procainamide
Myotonic syndrome	Propranolol

Note: Only drugs commonly used in the elderly are listed.

References

Ballantyne J (1970) Iatrogenic deafness. J Laryngol 84: 967–1000

Corrigan AB, Robinson RG, Terenty R, Dick-Smith JB, Walters D (1974) Benign rheumatoid arthritis of the aged. Br Med J 1: 444–446

Esselinckx W, Doherty SM, Dixon AS (1977) Polymyalgia rheumatica. Abrupt and gradual withdrawal of prednisolone treatment, clinical and laboratory observations. Ann Rheum Dis 36: 219–224

Grimley Evans J (1979) Fractured proximal femur in Newcastle upon Tyne. Age Ageing 8: 16–24

Inman WH (1977) Study of fatal bone marrow depression with special reference to phenylbutazone and oxphenbutazone. Br Med J 1: 1500–1505

Jones TG, Hazleman BL (1981) Prognosis and management of polymyalgia rheumatica. Ann Rheum Dis 40: 1–5

Jowsey J (1977) Osteoporosis: dealing with a crippling bone disease in the elderly. Geriatrics 32: 41–50

Scott JT (1977) Choice of treatment in gout. Practitioner 219: 469–489

9 Metabolic and Nutritional Disorders

Thyroid Disease

Diagnosis

Epidemiological studies correlating thyroid disease with ageing have been carried out over many years. From these studies it is clear that in old age mild degrees of hyperthyroidism due to an autonomous adenoma are more common than those due to Graves' disease. This contrasts with younger patients where thyrotoxicosis usually is due to the latter. There also is a group who have a multinodular goitre associated with autonomous function and high serum T3 concentrations. It may be that they have subclinical hyperthyroidism.

Originally it was thought that thyrotoxicosis was a disease of younger women, but currently the evidence is that around 40% of cases occur in patients over the age of 60 years. The prevalence of the disease in old people varies from 0.5% to 2.3% depending on the group studied. Misdiagnosis of the elderly thyrotoxic frequently occurs due to the atypical presentation of symptoms in those individuals. Again up to 40% of patients have no palpable thyroid tissue or goitre. The symptom particularly noticeable by its absence is that of tachycardia so prevalent in younger patients. In contrast, atrial fibrillation occurs in some 50% of elderly thyrotoxic patients. Symptoms often are vague and include anorexia and weight loss with associated lassitude. Occasionally patients become apathetic and may even be misdiagnosed as having hypothyroidism.

At the other extreme, myxoedema also is easily missed in the elderly. It must always be considered in patients with non-specific symptoms. Indeed there is a strong case for screening all elderly patients for the disorder. This applies not only to in-patients, but also to out-patients. Frequently the myxoedematous or hypothyroid patients appears at out-patient departments other than the endocrine clinic. Sometimes she presents at the ear, nose, and throat department with hoarseness of voice or deafness; at the neurological department with ataxia, paraesthesia, and neuropathies; at the gastro-intestinal department with constipation or diarrhoea; or as a general medical admission with increasing inability to cope at home.

Signs which are useful in the young patient, such as a coarse skin, thinning of scalp hair, and sluggish reflexes are less reliable in old age since ageing itself produces many of these. This further strengthens the case for routine screening.

There are clear advantages in diagnosing hypothyroidism before it becomes clinically advanced, as treatment of the established disease becomes increasingly hazardous even when exceptionally small dosages of replacement therapy are used. The prevalence of hypothyroidism varies in several studies from 0.8% to 1.1% in out-patient populations, increasing to 2% of in-patients in geriatric units.

Thyroid function tests in the elderly individual are often difficult to interpret in the presence of other disease processes. A diagnosis should not be made on the basis of an abnormal serum thyroxine concentration alone. Hypothyroidism should be confirmed by identifying a higher thyroid stimulating hormone concentration, and thyrotoxicosis by measuring a high serum tri-iodothyronine concentration.

Treatment and Management

Thyrotoxicosis

Radio-iodine is the most commonly used treatment of thyrotoxicosis in elderly patients. The factors that constrain its use in young patients such as genetic damage, carcinogenesis, and hypothyroidism are not applicable to the elderly. Hypothyroidism can follow the use of ^{131}I in the elderly as in the young, but the shorter life expectancy reduces the extent of the problem.

There is general agreement now that the effects of recurrent or inadequately treated thyrotoxicosis in the elderly are especially undesirable, particularly in those patients who have underlying cardiovascular disease. As a result slightly larger doses of ^{131}I are often administered than would be the case in younger patients, even though this increases the risk of subsequent hypothyroidism. Other antithyroid medication has to be stopped prior to and for 48 h following the administration of ^{131}I, but may be recommenced for a period of time until the radio-iodine has effectively eliminated the condition.

Hypothyroidism

The treatment of hypothyroidism in the elderly is essentially the same as that required for the treatment of hypothyroidism in the young, apart from the precaution that thyroxine should be commenced at lower dosages and increased more slowly than would normally be the case for younger individuals. An example is that if there is overt cardiac disease, the dose should be 50 μg on alternate days, increasing this no more frequently than at monthly intervals. A more rapid increase may precipitate angina or frank myocardial infarction.

Following commencement of therapy, frequent checks of thyroid function should be carried out to establish adequate replacement therapy. Since hypothyroidism may follow ^{131}I treatment for thyrotoxicosis, all patients managed in this way should have their thyroid function tests checked at regular intervals so as to prevent the later onset of clinical hypothyroidism. Some centres have a register of such patients, and it is wise that any patient treated with ^{131}I should be placed on this so that suitable follow-up can be arranged.

Myxoedema Coma

Myxoedema coma is characterised by exaggeration of the signs and symptoms of untreated hypothyroidism with increasing predominance of neurological symptoms, leading to impairment of consciousness, and eventually coma. Characteristically, the patient is an elderly female in whom the coma has been precipitated by infection, drugs, hypothermia, or a cardiovascular accident, e.g. myocardial infarction or cerebrovascular accident. Mortality is very high at between 60% and 70%, depending on the study examined. Inadequate control of the precipitating factors or complications is the prime reason for the high mortality. Severe hypothermia delays initiating therapy and inadequate doses of thyroid replacement are often given.

Treatment comprises the administration of thyroid hormones, administration of glucocorticoids, correction of hypothermia, and correction of the electrolyte disturbances, particularly hyponatraemia by fluid restriction. There also should be adequate treatment of the precipitating cause. Following intravenous administration of tri-iodothyronine (at 100 μg followed by 25 μg six-hourly) a therapeutic response is usually seen within the first 24 h. Thereafter the patient can be prescribed oral thyroid replacement. Steroid therapy in a dose of 100 mg hydrocortisone intravenously six-hourly is administered so as to cover the possibility of adrenal crisis, particularly as it is often difficult to distinguish primary from secondary hypothyroidism.

A note of caution must be sounded in the correction of the hypothermia, for if too rapid reheating occurs there is risk of coma arising because blood supplying vital organs such as the brain, heart, and lungs is diverted to the periphery. Correction of carbon dioxide retention is usually easily accomplished either by oxygen administration or, where necessary, assistance using the respirator.

Myxoedema coma has a high mortality because in the majority of cases there is a failure to recognise the underlying myxoedematous state. It is often mistaken for other diseases.

Diabetes Mellitus

Diagnosis

Diabetes mellitus is one of the most common diseases among older people, affecting 17% of those over 65 years and 26% of those over 85. Its prevalence amongst older people is rising steadily, probably as a result of increasing obesity, an increase in longevity, and better methods for detecting the condition. Despite increased awareness, however, a large number of elderly diabetics go undiagnosed for considerable lengths of time.

Glucose tolerance decreases with age to the extent that approximately 50% of the population over the age of 70 have an abnormal blood glucose at 1–2 h after a meal. The change is progressive, giving rise to a steady decline in glucose tolerance from the age of 50 onwards. The mechanism for this is unclear. Several studies have given conflicting results. Such mechanisms as decreased insulin release and decreased sensitivity to insulin have been postulated. Clearly, if glucose tolerance generally decreases with age then diagnosis of diabetes mellitus in the elderly becomes increasingly difficult, particularly if the same criteria are used as those applied to younger individuals. Some workers have suggested that diabetes mellitus should be diagnosed on the basis of a fasting blood glucose rather than a glucose tolerance test.

Diagnosis of diabetes mellitus in older people should be made if at any time fasting hyperglycaemia is found or if the elderly patient has symptoms consistent with the diagnosis of diabetes, even when fasting glucose levels are borderline. These individuals should be subjected to an oral glucose tolerance test to confirm the diagnosis, leading in turn to appropriate therapy.

Any elderly patient who has obesity of greater than 20% above the ideal body weight or evidence of cerebral, coronary, or peripheral vascular disease should be screened for diabetes mellitus. This can be completely asymptomatic in the elderly, particularly in the early period, when it may be confused for other diseases. Mild to moderate hyperglycaemia without acidosis is the common presenting feature of the disease in the elderly, usually in the obese. This may result from a tissue resistance to insulin rather than to absolute insulin deficiency. The first symptoms may be manifestation of complications such as neuropathy, impotence, recurrent urinary tract infection, myopathy, or vascular episodes.

Treatment

Treatment of diabetes mellitus in the elderly is based on either diet alone, or diet and oral hypoglycaemic, or diet and insulin therapy, depending on the severity of the condition. Often its onset is insidious, during which time the elderly patient may become severely hyperglycaemic and dehydrated, developing hyperosmolar non-ketotic coma as its first manifestation. This serious, frequently fatal complication warrants special attention in a discussion of diabetes in the elderly.

The vascular and neuropathic complications deteriorate in patients with poor diabetic control. Treatment should therefore be aimed at maintaining the diabetic in as normal a metabolic state as possible. Increasing age and duration of diabetes increase the frequency with which errors in medication occur, leading in turn to an increased morbidity.

Proper foot care is particularly important in older diabetics, because of the increase of injury that occurs both with forgetfulness and failing eyesight in association with poor or deteriorating vascular status and neuropathic status. All older diabetic patients should be seen by a chiropodist periodically for care of the nails and calluses and guidance to proper footwear so that many of the vascular and infective complications can be avoided.

Emergency Treatment

Hyperosmolar Non-ketotic Coma

The typical presentation is of progressive hyperglycaemia leading to dehydration which in turn may progress to shock, confusion and coma. The plasma glucose usually is exceedingly high; serum osmolality is high; serum sodium is often, but not invariably, elevated; and the serum potassium may or may not be normal. The pathogenesis of the syndrome is not entirely clearly understood, but it is believed that patients who develop it produce enough insulin to minimise lipolysis. This prevents development of ketoacidosis, but does not control hyperglycaemia with consequent hyperosmolality.

Some 5%–10% of the hyperglycaemic comas in the total population are of the hyperosmolar-hyperglycaemic non-ketotic type. The prevalence rises with increasing age. Immediate goals of therapy are correction of dehydration through administration of appropriate fluid and correction of hyperglycaemia through the use of insulin. Relief of fluid depletion and administration of insulin must be accomplished cautiously, precisely, and slowly in a setting where constant monitoring of the central venous pressure and of blood glucose, urea, and electrolytes is possible.

Fluid should be given with intravenous normal saline to restore the extracellular intravascular volume, even though the ultimate replacement of the fluid deficit will require water in excess of salt. If the patient is shocked, then plasma blood volume expanders should be used initially. When vital signs are stable, isotonic saline should be changed to hypotonic saline to correct the hypernatraemia. Fluid replacement should continue at a rate aimed at achieving approximately half the estimated amount needed to restore normal body fluid volumes within the first 24 h. Insulin should be given by either the intravenous or the intramuscular route, with the plasma glucose level being determined hourly. Subcutaneous insulin should not be prescribed in this situation as a poor circulation makes absorption inconsistent. Since a patient with non-ketotic hyperglycaemia requires less insulin than one with a ketoacidosis, he should be carefully monitored for impending hypoglycaemia.

Heparin is often used to prevent the late onset of thrombotic episodes and reduce the incidence of disseminated intravascular coagulation. Following the control of the hyperosmolar coma, patients can be satisfactorily controlled on either diet alone or diet plus oral hypoglycaemic agents; only a small proportion require continued insulin therapy.

Hyperglycaemic Ketoacidosis

Severe hyperglycaemic ketoacidosis has a mortality rate of 5%–10% in the young population. In old age the condition carries considerably higher mortality, which approaches 50% in most centres. It should be managed along lines appropriate for younger individuals. Special points are that a central venous pressure line should be inserted as a useful guide to fluid therapy, particularly in those patients who have underlying cardiovascular disease. Subcutaneous heparin also should be used, particularly in individuals who are hyperosmolar and unconscious, unless there are obvious contraindications. Ketoacidosis usually occurs in diabetics whose insulin is inadequate to prevent lipolysis and in those previously known to be on insulin.

Hypoglycaemic Coma

This is most commonly seen in those who are insulin-dependent and is the most frequent reason for impaired consciousness in the diabetic taking insulin. Hypoglycaemia can also occur in patients taking sulphonylureas, though this is less common than the coma produced by insulin.

If the patient is unconscious, intravenous glucose is mandatory using 50 ml of 50% dextrose in the first instance to see if this can reverse the coma. It is not uncommon for the elderly individual who has suffered a hypoglycaemic coma to be confused for a considerable time after correction of his hypoglycaemic state, and the patient may have to be kept in hospital until this has resolved.

Lactic Acidosis

Lactic acidosis is a rare side-effect of the biguanides when they are used in the elderly population. As a result phenformin and the other biguanides have been used less frequently, so that the condition is becoming increasingly rare. Lactic acidosis is difficult to treat and often resistant to therapy. Large amounts of bicarbonate are often needed to treat the acidosis and, if it is particularly severe, dialysis may be required. Clearly, if a drug is thought to be responsible it should be stopped.

Maintenance Therapy

Diet

In the elderly, diabetes often is diagnosed with the detection of glycosuria on a randomly taken urine specimen or hyperglycaemia on a random sample of blood. The majority of these individuals can be satisfactorily controlled with the use of dietary advice and only a smaller percentage require to take oral hypoglycaemic agents. An even smaller minority require insulin therapy. Weight reduction often is all that is needed.

Oral Hypoglycaemic Agents

There continues to be controversy about the usefulness and the safety of the currently available oral hypoglycaemic agents, particularly in the report from the National Commission on Diabetes. This reported an increased mortality in individuals taking oral hypoglycaemic agents, particularly amongst those with coexisting cardiovascular disease. Prior to prescribing an agent, the benefits and risks must be weighed up so that the best treatment for the individual patient can be obtained.

Sulphonylureas. The sulphonylureas act mainly by augmenting insulin secretion and consequently are effective only when some residual pancreatic beta-cell activity is present. They should only be used after a failure to respond to a suitable diet for a period of time, and should complement rather than replace the diet. In the United Kingdom, tolbutamide, chlorpropamide, and glibenclamide are the most commonly used agents. There are advantages in using a shorter-acting oral hypoglycaemic agent, such as tolbutamide or glipizide in old age. The longer-acting agents may cause prolonged hypoglycaemia in patients who have underlying renal impairment. Sulphonylureas are contraindicated in patients who are particularly obese until their body weight has fallen to within 15% of their ideal body weight, or where the diabetes has not been controlled by simpler measures.

Adverse reactions of the sulphonylureas are common and are similar to those of sulphonamides in general. These include hypothyroidism, abnormalities of liver function, and haematological disorders. If renal function is impaired, both glibenclamide and glipizide have unchanged half-lives, whereas chlorpropamide and tolbutamide have markedly prolonged ones. Individual sulphonylureas are discussed below.

Chlorpropamide is considered as having the highest incidence of toxic effects amongst the sulphonylureas. The explanation for this probably is that a large number of patients are given high doses and that this increases the probability of adverse reactions. It is eliminated by excretion from the kidneys, so that cumulation occurs in patients who have renal tubular dysfunction. Hypoglycaemia caused by chlorpropamide may be prolonged and is not always correlated to the blood levels of the drug or with increased levels of insulin. Therefore, since elderly patients often have poor renal function they should not be given chlorpropamide.

A further problem is that chlorpropamide sometimes induces the syndrome of inappropriate antidiuretic hormone secretion. The symptoms are similar to water intoxication and consist of confusion, nausea, dizziness, anorexia, and depression. Elderly patients seem to be at a higher risk from this complication. In cardiac failure the problem may manifest itself as a poor response to diuretic therapy.

Tolbutamide is one of the oldest and one of the least toxic sulphonylureas. Side-effects occur in less than 1.5% of all treated patients. Some long-term studies appear to suggest that there may be an increased cardiovascular mortality, but many people have reservations about the interpretation of these reports. Tolbutamide is less likely to cause hypoglycaemia than the newer more potent sulphonylureas. An exception is in renal failure, where its half-life is prolonged and the risk of hypoglycaemia increased unless dosage is reduced.

The absorption of *glibenclamide* is variable and irregular in individual patients. Its duration of action is between that of chlorpropamide and tolbutamide. A particular feature of glibenclamide is that, after some weeks of treatment, plasma insulin levels rise so that its dose has to be reduced.

Glipizide is almost as potent as glibenclamide, but is absorbed rapidly and has a relatively short half-life. It is primarily metabolised by the liver. Side-effects occur in 7%–8% of patients. An advantage is that it does not produce the prolonged effects of drugs such as chlorpropamide and that its dose can be titrated throughout the day according to the individual needs.

The Biguanides.   The biguanides metformin and phenformin act by interfering with glucose transport through the intestinal mucosa and inhibition of gluconeogenesis, fatty acid oxidation, and lipid synthesis. Metformin, the only biguanide still commonly used, is absorbed completely after oral administration. The most dangerous side-effect of the biguanides, particularly phenformin, is lactic acidosis, which, when it occurs, is lethal in approximately 50% of cases. Metformin is less likely to cause this so that it is still used either alone or with a sulphonylurea in the overweight diabetic who cannot be adequately controlled with diet alone. A further problem is that biguanides cause gastrointestinal disturbances in approximately 25% of patients. Metformin should not be prescribed if there is renal failure, respiratory insufficiency, cirrhosis of the liver, hepatitis, alcoholism, or addiction, nor in pre- and postoperative states. In these situations clearance of the drug is diminished, so that the risk of toxicity is increased.

There is no difference in the use of *insulin* in an elderly insulin-dependent diabetic from that in a younger one. When failing eyesight or early dementia occurs, arrangements should be made for a willing relative or district nurse to come and administer the insulin. This reduces the risk of accidental over- or underdosage. Mealtimes tend to be erratic and often contain foods inappropriate to the needs of the insulin-dependent diabetic. Close monitoring of diet therefore is important.

Nutrition

Our knowledge of the nutritional needs of adults has been based mainly on studies of young adults, the needs of the elderly being largely estimated by extrapolation of the results seen in this group. The intakes of energy, protein, minerals, and vitamins all decline with age in healthy individuals. This usually follows a decline in energy expenditure and thus does not result in weight loss or subnutrition. Likewise, the age-related decline in skeletal mass probably is the cause rather than the result of a reduced protein intake.

Subnutrition

In old age, subnutrition occurs mainly in patients whose mental and physical impairment prevents them from obtaining, preparing, and eating food. If an individual is healthy neither social isolation nor a low income have a serious effect on food intake. Estimates from the Department of Health and Social Security suggest that 6% of men and 5% of women between the ages of 70 and 80 years and 12% of men and 8% of women over 80 years of age are suffering from one or more forms of subnutrition. Commonly these consist of protein-energy malnutrition or deficiency of iron, potassium, thiamine, pyridoxine, nicotinic acid, folic acid, ascorbic acid, or vitamin D. Old people who are housebound face the additional problem of not receiving sufficient sunlight to convert subcutaneous 7-dihydrotachysterol into vitamin D.

Treatment of malnutrition depends upon the identification of old people most at risk. These include patients recently bereaved or recently discharged from hospital who are known to suffer from severe mental or physical incapacity. Nutrition often can be improved by sending in a home help or by inviting the patient to a day centre, a day hospital, or a luncheon club. A meals-on-wheels service also may help. However, this only is effective if it provides meals at least 5 days a week, if the patient actually eats them, and if care has been taken to avoid destruction of ascorbic and folic acids during their preparation.

If such measures fail to maintain nutrition, mineral and vitamin supplements should be considered. Many old people have a low intake of potassium, but it is only those who are on diuretics who require supplements (Chap. 3). Most old people take adequate quantities of calcium, but there may be a case for giving supplements to those with osteoporosis (Chap. 8).

Thiamine, nicotinic acid, pyridoxine, and riboflavine deficiencies are common in sick old people. However, the correlation is poor between low blood levels of these and clinical signs such as glossitis, stomatitis, neuropathy, cardiac failure, or mental impairment. Such signs more usually are due to disorders coincidental to the deficiency. Some clinicians use parenteral injections of B vitamins in acutely confused old people. An example is strong vitamin B and C injections given in a dose of 7 ml daily for 10 days. There is no objective evidence, however, that such a regime actually works.

Even healthy old people may have low intakes of ascorbic acid. This probably relates to the cost of fruit and fresh vegetables. The problem is even greater in ill health where the patient is unable to purchase or prepare food. There is the additional factor that leucocyte ascorbic acid levels are suppressed by traumatic, ischaemic, malignant, or inflammatory conditions. Here doses of up to 2 g/day of the vitamin may be insufficient to correct blood levels. There is no evidence that in these situations a temporary reduction in ascorbic acid concentrations causes harm or that correction with large doses of vitamin has any effect on outcome.

A wide range of effects has been claimed for ascorbic acid, but the only one of proven importance is that it improves the rate of healing of surgical wounds, pressure areas, and varicose ulcers. Here a dose of 200 mg daily is more than adequate.

The vitamin also may reduce the symptoms of the common cold, but does not prevent the infection. Again, there is circumstantial evidence that if patients are taking aspirin, ascorbic acid supplements may reduce the amount of gastrointestinal haemorrhage. Occasionally, patients present with the classical picture of scurvy, but this is rare. There is speculation that ascorbic acid may be responsible for the weakness, depression, tiredness, and reduced resistance to infection found in frail old people, but there is no firm evidence to back this up.

Massive doses of ascorbic acid have been advocated in the treatment of such diverse conditions as atherosclerosis and carcinomatosis. There is no practical or theoretical justification for such an approach. Large doses, in fact, may cause diarrhoea. There is the additional problem that they increase the rate of ascorbic acid metabolism, so that when they are stopped, frank scurvy may be precipitated.

Obesity

The causes of obesity are obscure, relating to both an increased energy intake and a change in metabolism. In old age the relationship between intake and body build is poor, so that many obese old women have an energy intake as low as 1000 calories. This may be due to the fact that limited mobility reduces energy expenditure, and that obesity insulates against energy being lost as heat.

The only effective way of achieving weight reduction is to reduce the calorie intake. Since the intake of many obese patients is already low, effective weight loss sometimes only is achieved by restricting this to as little as 600 calories per day. At this level it is difficult to provide a balanced diet, so that iron and vitamin B, C, and D supplements should be added.

Old people should not be given appetite suppressants. They have little efficacy and often produce severe side-effects. Fenfluramine, for example, often causes drowsiness and confusion. Changes in affect and paranoid episodes have also been reported. Withdrawal also is a problem, in that it may precipitate severe depression.

Anaemia

Iron Deficiency

Even healthy old people have low intakes of iron. Surprisingly, however, dietary deficiency rarely causes iron-deficiency anaemia. This condition more commonly is the result of blood loss either from alimentary lesions or from treatment with non-steroidal anti-inflammatory agents (Chap. 8). It is important, therefore, that the cause of the anaemia be investigated before supplements are started.

Most elderly patients can be treated adequately with ferrous sulphate in a dose of 200 mg three times per day. The main side-effect is gastro-intestinal intolerance with nausea, vomiting, diarrhoea, or constipation. If these occur, other preparations such as slow-release ferrous sulphate may be tried. Another argument for using slow-release preparations is that they are only taken once a day. However, old people are able to absorb only 60 mg of elemental iron per day, so that a once a day dose of ferrous sulphate would probably be adequate in a patient who had compliance problems.

Iron also may be given parenterally. Since intra-muscular iron injections are painful and old people often have gross muscle atrophy, the element should be given intravenously. The main reason for using this route is to correct iron depletion if it seems unlikely that a patient will take an oral preparation when he goes home. Before resorting to it, however, the physician should be convinced that correction of the iron deficiency is really necessary and should already have tried the patient on tablets. Intravenous iron rarely causes problems, but occasionally produces a serious anaphylactic reaction. It should only be used in exceptional circumstances, therefore.

Many non-anaemia patients have a low serum iron concentration. Since many old women are tired, feel dizzy, are breathless and weak, and feel irritable, there is the temptation to attribute these symptoms to iron deficiency and to treat them with supplements. There is no evidence that this does any good. In fact, old women with a mild iron-deficiency anaemia have a greater life expectancy than their non-anaemic counterparts.

A more appropriate approach is to recognise that iron deficiency is indicative of underlying disease and to search for this. Iron supplements are only likely to benefit the patient if, in addition to having iron deficiency, he also has a severe anaemia (say a haemoglobin of less than 10 g/dl).

Folic Acid Deficiency

The prevalence of this varies in different groups of old people and in different parts of the United Kingdom. It is particularly common in patients who have severe mental and physical incapacity and who have difficulty in nourishing themselves, but is rare in healthy old people even if they have a low income and are living alone.

Folic acid deficiency may give rise to neurological abnormalities similar to those related to B_{12} deficiency. They include mental impairment and signs of a myelopathy and peripheral neuropathy. Treatment with supplements may produce a dramatic improvement. Many demented patients suffer from folic acid deficiency, but few of them show benefit from supplements. This is because, in most instances, folic acid is the result and not the cause of mental impairment.

Folic-acid-deficiency anaemia should be treated with folic acid tablets in a dose of 10–20 mg daily, reducing this to a maintenance dose of 2.5–10 mg daily once the haemoglobin has returned to normal.

Although every undergraduate knows that folic acid should not be given to a patient with B_{12} deficiency, this continues to happen all too frequently in practice. Often this is due to a doctor paying insufficient attention to the contents of a compound haematinic tablet or multivitamin preparation.

Vitamin B_{12} Deficiency

This usually is due to a failure of intrinsic factor secretion associated with atrophic gastritis. Other important causes in old age are bacterial overgrowth in the small bowel associated with a Billroth II gastrectomy, or jejunal diverticular disease. Dietary deficiency of the vitamin is rare.

Treatment is with intramuscular cyanocobalamin 1000 μg weekly for 4 weeks, followed by a maintenance dose of 250 μg every month. Hydroxycobalamin has a stronger affinity for albumin and is excreted more slowly. It may be given less frequently and in smaller doses than cyanocobalamin. Its advantages, however, are theoretical rather than practical.

Further Reading

Burroughs V, Shenkman L (1982) Thyroid function in the elderly. Am J Med Sci 283: 8–17
Green M (1981) Ageing and disease. Clin Endocrinol Metab 10: 207–228
Harvard CW (1981) The thyroid and ageing. Clin Endocrinol Metab 10: 163–178
Williams TF (1981) Diabetes mellitus. Clin Endocrinol Metab 10: 179–194

Cerebrovascular Disease

Prevention

In cerebrovascular disease a high serum cholesterol and cigarette smoking only have a marginal effect on the incidence of atherothrombotic brain infarction. Glucose intolerance is more important, and it is likely that effective control of blood glucose concentrations would reduce substantially the incidence of strokes in elderly diabetics. The influence of hypertension, however, predominates, and increases with the age of the patient (Fig. 10.1). It would appear reasonable, therefore, that treatment aimed at reducing hypertension would reduce the risk of a stroke. Long-term studies are in progress at present to confirm or refute this hypothesis. In the meantime, most clinicians feel justified in treating a high blood pressure in old age (Chap. 4).

Patients with atrial fibrillation are at increased risk from cerebral embolism. In the Framingham study subjects with atrial fibrillation had almost six times the risk of developing a stroke compared with the rest of the population (Kannel et al. 1978). The duration of the arrhythmia is unimportant, so that the patient who has had atrial fibrillation for 10 years is as likely to have a stroke as one who has had the condition for 10 days. This raises the question as to whether patients with atrial fibrillation should be treated with anticoagulants. Most authorities answer in the affirmative (Millikan 1979). Despite this, many patients with atrial fibrillation discharged from geriatric units or attending day hospitals are not on this treatment, suggesting that most clinicians believe that the risks of poor compliance or drug interactions outweigh theoretical benefits. An investigation into the clincial justification for this approach is required.

The earliest warning of impending cerebrovascular damage may be a transient ischaemic attack, in which focal neurological signs occur suddenly but resolve within 24 h. This commonly is due to an area of stenosis in a carotid artery from which clumps of platelets break off to block the distal arterial tree (Marshall 1976). Platelet emboli also may have their origin from damaged mitral or aortic valve cusps.

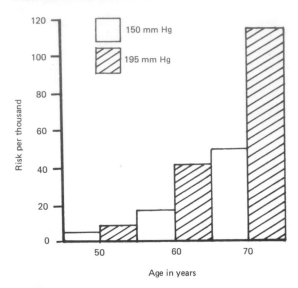

Fig. 10.1. Risk of atherothrombotic brain infarction in women with systolic pressures of 150 and 195 mm Hg (Kannel et al. 1978).

In view of the fact that transient ischaemic attacks usually are followed ultimately by a completed stroke, a great deal of attention has been given to devising means to prevent the formation of platelet thrombi. This may be done by using agents which block the formation of thromboxane A_2, a prostaglandin with a powerful aggregating effect on platelets and produced by platelets themselves. In physiological situations the effect of thromboxane A_2 is balanced by prostacyclin, a desegregating agent produced by the blood vessel wall (Fig. 10.2).

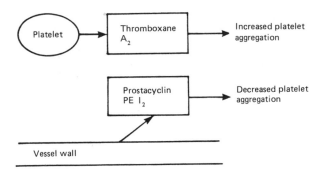

Fig. 10.2. Factors affecting platelet aggregation.

Aspirin blocks the action of cyclo-oxygenase, the enzyme responsible for the formation of both thromboxane A_2 and prostacyclin. In small doses, however, it suppresses the former without affecting the latter. In clinical practice, it has proven extremely difficult to give the correct dose to achieve the desired effect. In one study, aspirin in a dose of 1300 mg daily reduced the incidence of transient ischaemic attacks but did not prevent stroke formation (Fields 1979). Another showed that 325 mg aspirin four times a day produced a 19% reduction in the incidence of transient ischaemic attacks and a 31% reduction in that of strokes. The vasodilator dipyridamole and the uricosuric agent sulphin-pyrazone also inhibit platelet aggregation. Despite this in vitro effect, sulphin-pyrazone either alone or in combination with aspirin has no effect on the incidence of transient ischaemic attacks or strokes (Canadian Cooperative Study Group 1978). Dipyridamole when given alone also has no effect on transient ischaemic attacks (Acheson et al. 1969). Further work is required to establish whether the probable synergism between dipyridamole and aspirin is of clinical relevance. At present, however, the most rational approach to preventing platelet aggregation would appear to be to give 325 mg aspirin four times daily.

An alternative is to prevent intra-arterial thrombosis using anticoagulants. This initially produces a marginal reduction in the incidence of completed strokes, but the effect is not maintained beyond 3–6 months (Mitchell 1979).

It should be recognised of course that only a proportion of transient ischaemic attacks are due to platelet embolism. Hypertension and transient arrhythmias may also cause these episodes and should be diagnosed and treated appropriately (Chap. 4).

Treatment of Acute Stroke

The initial management of a cerebrovascular accident consists of ensuring that the airway is patent, that hydration and nutrition are adequate, that pressure areas are avoided, and that respiratory infections are controlled. Attention may also be directed at minimising the extent of cerebrovascular damage.

Intervention seems particularly appropriate if there is continuing progression in neurological damage (stroke in evolution). This pattern usually reflects extension of thrombosis within the cerebral blood vessels, and the prompt administration of anticoagulants reduces the extent of cerebral damage. The usual regime is to start with intravenous heparin and to continue with a coumarin anticoagulant for up to 3 months (Chap. 3). Such an approach will be disastrous if the lesion is a cerebral haemorrhage, so treatment should be preceded by a lumbar puncture to check for blood in the cerebrospinal fluid. A preferable alternative is to use computerised tomography if this is available and can be performed quickly enough.

Deterioration in clinical signs also may be the result of cerebral oedema, and a variety of agents have been tried to prevent this happening. One of these is 20% mannitol. This acts by increasing serum osmolarity so that water is drawn from the brain into the bloodstream. A typical dose would be 1 g mannitol/kg body weight given over 10 minutes. Though this approach is useful in some forms of cerebral oedema it is of little value in cerebrovascular disease. This is possibly because areas of infarction have high permeability, so that mannitol simply leaks into the damaged tissues where it is unable to exert its osmotic effect. Dextran 40 is another material which increases the osmolarity of plasma. In acute stroke it may be given in a dose of 500 ml 10% solution over 1 h followed by 500 ml 12-hourly for 72 h. This may reduce initial mortality in severe strokes, but has no effect on long-term disability. Alternative hypertonic solutions are isosorbide and glycerol, but these have proven of little value in cerebrovascular disease.

Another way of reducing oedema is to use corticosteroids. Their precise mode of action is unclear, but they are extremely effective in removing fluid from oedematous areas of the brain. If dexamethasone is used its dosage is in the order of 4 mg six-hourly. Unfortunately, this approach has little effect on the outcome of a stroke in terms of function or mortality.

Patients with acute strokes also have been treated with agents designed to improve the metabolism of surviving neurones. Naftidrofuryl increases the oxidative metabolism of tissues by activating succinic dehydrogenase, a tricarboxylic acid cycle enzyme, and thus has theoretical advantages in situations such as cerebrovascular disease where there is anoxia. In one trial, patients with an acute stroke on 200 mg naftidrofuryl three times daily had a lower mortality and a higher discharge rate than controls on a placebo (Admani 1978). Further work is required to confirm or refute the value of such an approach.

Prevention of Recurrence

Once the condition of a patient has stabilised, attention should be directed to preventing a recurrence. Even after a completed stroke, effective control of hypertension reduces the frequency of further episodes and increases life expectancy. It must be recognised, however, that patients with cerebrovascular disease lose the ability to regulate cerebral blood flow in response to hypotension. A sudden fall in blood pressure thus may cut off the supply of blood from ischaemic areas. Caution is vital when treating hypertension in this situation.

Attempts have been made to reduce the recurrence of cerebral thrombosis by using anticoagulants. Any reduction in thrombosis, however, is balanced by an increased incidence of cerebral haemorrhage. Though antiplatelet agents may be useful in transient ischaemic attacks, there is little place for them once a stroke has been established.

Treatment of Stroke Disability

Recovery of function after a stroke is dependent primarily on the skill and hard work of the physiotherapist, occupational therapist, nurse, and patient himself, and drug treatment only has a minor role to play in this situation. The main contribution drugs can make is in the relief of spasticity. Situations in which increased tone may create difficulty are elbow flexion interfering with dressing, or plantar flexion interfering with walking. Unfortunately, spasmolytic drugs are not selective in their action. They may relieve plantar flexion at the expense of the beneficial effect which spasticity has in bracing a knee joint in extension. The best approach to spasticity, then, is to re-educate weak muscles so that contraction of one group does not invariably result in excessive contraction of antagonists. Muscle relaxants should be used only as an adjunct to such treatment.

The most widely used muscle relaxant is diazepam. This has a non-specific effect on the many synapses involved in motor function in the brainstem and spinal cord. Its sedative effects on the cerebral cortex provide an important additional source of muscle relaxation. Doses of between 2 mg and 5 mg three times daily are required to produce the desired effect. It may also be used in a dose of 10 mg intramuscularly to relieve an acute episode of spasm or, occasionally, to prepare for a session of passive physiotherapy. In old age, a dose large enough to achieve significant muscle relaxation often is accompanied by intolerable side-effects. The patient may simply fall asleep, or become confused and disinhibited. Coordination also may be impaired, seriously compromising attempts at mobilisation. Chlordiazepoxide is an alternative to diazepam with the same potency and the same drawbacks.

Baclofen has a specific effect on the afferent-efferent synapses for motor units within the spinal cord. It has been widely used in the treatment of spasticity associated with damage to the spinal cord. More recently it has been shown to reduce tone and to improve mobility in patients recovering from strokes. Side-effects include sedation and vertigo and, less commonly, euphoria, depression, confusion, or hallucinations. Further experience is required to evaluate whether these difficulties pose major problems in the elderly.

Dantrolene has a more direct muscle relaxant effect, in which it suppresses the release of calcium from the sarcoplasmic reticulum, thus inhibiting the interaction of thick and thin filaments to cause muscle contraction. It is effective in relieving spasticity due to spinal cord injury, stroke, cerebral palsy, and multiple sclerosis. The initial oral dose is 25 mg/day increasing by 25 mg every 4–7 days to a maximum of 100 mg three times daily. Despite its peripheral site of action the drug can cause drowsiness or dizziness. A more serious problem is that of hepatitis, occurring in 0.35%–0.5% of patients on treatment for more than 60 days. A regular review of liver function tests is essential.

Many patients with cerebrovascular disease have limb pain. This may be due to joint adhesions (e.g. frozen shoulder), to muscle spasm, or to thalamic damage with causalgia. Treatment includes physiotherapy, muscle relaxants, and analgesics. In a few instances, intermittent episodes of limb pain are related to sensory epilepsy. This may be missed in that there may be no other symptoms. A trial of phenytoin or carbamezapine is worthwhile in these circumstances.

Cerebrovascular disease often is accompanied by depression. This frequently responds to tricyclic antidepressants, but in view of the fact that strokes are often accompanied by cardiovascular damage it may be wise to avoid more cardiotoxic agents, such as imipramine and amitriptyline, using others such as mianserin, doxepin, nomifensine, or maprotiline (Chap. 12). Patients with multiple cerebral infarcts may have mental impairment. Cerebral vasodilators are useless in this situation (Chap. 12).

Parkinson's Disease

Modern drug developments have revolutionised the management of this disorder. A prerequisite to an effective response, however, is that the diagnosis should be accurate. Many old people treated with anti-Parkinsonian drugs have rigidity and akinesia related to generalised cerebral damage rather than to changes in the basal nuclei and substantia nigra. Such people do not respond to treatment and may often be severely incapacitated by side-effects. The distinction from Parkinson's disease may be made by the absence of tremor and the presence of severe mental impairment. Mental impairment can occur in Parkinson's disease, but develops later on at an advanced stage of physical disability.

Anticholinergic Drugs

These act by preventing the uptake of acetylcholine by receptors in the basal nuclei, and thus redress the imbalance between acetylcholine and dopamine. A wide range is available (Table 10.1). They were for many years the mainstay of treatment in Parkinson's disease, but compared with levodopa they only have a minor effect on tremor, rigidity, and akinesia and have increasingly been replaced by the latter (White and Barnes 1981). Apart from their limited efficacy, anticholinergics have serious side-effects which are particularly troublesome in the elderly (Table 10.2). A further problem is that Parkinson's disease is

Table 10.1. Anticholinergic drugs available for treatment of Parkinson's disease

Benzpryzine
Benzhexol
Benztropine
Biperiden
Chlorphenoxamine
Cyclizine
Ethopropazine
Methixcine
Orphenadrine
Procyclidine

Table 10.1. Side-effects of anticholinergic
drugs of importance in the elderly

Drowsiness
Confusion
Hallucinations
Restlessness
Blurred vision
Precipitation of glaucoma
Constipation
Hypothermia
Postural hypotension
Urinary retention

accompanied by autonomic degeneration. This increases the risk of alimentary obstruction, urinary retention, hypothermia, and postural hypotension. The only place where anticholinergics have retained a major role is in the management of phenothiazine-induced Parkinsonism, where the unpredictable effect of levodopa gives cause for concern. Orphenadrine, by virtue of its mild euphoriant effect is the drug of choice in this situation. It can, however, cause serious oversedation.

Levodopa

This agent was introduced following the observation that in patients with Parkinson's disease, concentrations of dopamine were reduced in the basal nuclei and substantia nigra. It is absorbed from the gut and then penetrates the blood-brain barrier, where decarboxylase enzymes break it down to release dopamine. Replacement of dopamine produces an improvement in akinesia, rigidity, and tremor. In an early study a substantial improvement was found in half the patients and a moderate improvement in a quarter (Calne et al. 1969). The remaining quarter showed little change. Improvement may be sustained for a long time, so that after 6 years half the patients responding initially to levodopa can expect to be better than they were before the start of treatment (Shaw et al. 1980). Patients responding to treatment have a normal life expectancy, whereas those failing to respond or left untreated show a death rate which is twice to three times that of a control population. Despite the major impact that levodopa has had on the treatment of Parkinson's disease, it must be recognised that it does not arrest the natural progress of the disease. It merely postpones an inevitable deterioration in function by several years. In old people, the drug often postpones deterioration long enough to allow them to die from an unrelated condition before they become severely disabled.

Levodopa has a wide range of side-effects. The most prominent are nausea and anorexia (Fig. 10.3). This effect is related to stimulation of medullary

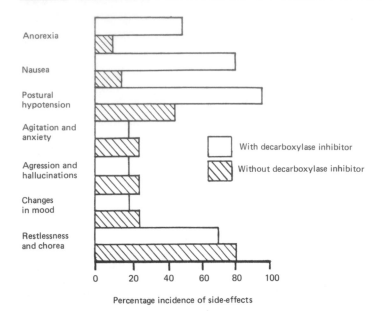

Anorexia

Nausea

Postural
hypotension

Agitation and
anxiety

□ With decarboxylase inhibitor

▨ Without decarboxylase inhibitor

Agression and
hallucinations

Changes
in mood

Restlessness
and chorea

0   20   40   60   80   100

Percentage incidence of side-effects

Fig. 10.3. Incidence of side-effects in patients receiving levodopa with and without decarboxylase inhibitor (Parkes 1981).

receptors rather than local gastro-intestinal irritation. It can be avoided by reducing the concentration of levodopa reaching these centres. This is done by giving the drug along with a decarboxylase inhibitor. It inhibits the formation of dopamine in the medulla, but because it does not penetrate the extrapyramidal centre, has no effect on dopamine concentrations at this site. The two decarboxylase inhibitors currently prepared in combination with levodopa are carbidopa and benserazide.

Another troublesome side-effect is postural hypotension. This is related to stimulation of blood vessels, nerve endings, and the midbrain. Fortunately in most patients the disorder does not produce symptoms. If it is troublesome it should be treated by changing the sleeping posture, using elastic stockings, or giving fludrocortisone.

Levodopa also occasionally causes cardiac arrhythmias. Despite the fact that old people, by virtue of multiple pathology, are at particular risk from these, the major benefits of levodopa far outweight this potential hazard.

About a quarter of patients on levodopa experience a variety of psychiatric disturbances. These include drowsiness, depression, anxiety, insomnia, nightmares, confusion, agitation, and hallucinations. The drug has to be given with particular care to old people with a previous history of depression or with evidence of chronic brain failure. There has been some suggestion that levodopa may sometimes cause a progressive and irreversible decline in mental function in some old people, but the evidence for this is unconvincing. It probably relates to the drug being used in patients coincidentally having a rapidly deteriorating dementia.

Although the psychiatric effects of levodopa usually are adverse it may occasionally improve mental function. An example is that it has been used in demented patients with low levels of dopamine in their cerebrospinal fluid. However, its activity is so unpredictable that it is unlikely ever to have a major role in the treatment of dementia. A more common benefit is that levodopa often has a mild euphoriant effect. This is useful in a disease which is associated with a very high incidence of depression.

Since alimentary, gastro-intestinal, and psychiatric side-effects are particularly common in old people, levodopa should be started at a very low dosage, and increased gradually, monitoring closely for symptoms. An example would be to start with Madopar (levodopa and benserazide) at 62.5 mg increasing by 62.5 mg every 3 days until maximum benefit has been achieved. The stage in the disease at which levodopa should be introduced also may be important. There is speculation that the earlier the drug is used, the sooner the patient will become refractory to it. The hypothesis is difficult to prove, but commonsense suggests that a drug with potentially serious side-effects should be withheld until the disease is having an important effect on a patient's daily activities.

Patients on levodopa frequently develop writhing movements of their lips and tongues. This is due to excessive quantities of dopamine in the corpus striatum, and indicates that the dose of levodopa is too large. The simplest solution is to reduce the dose. The movements may show a variety of cyclical patterns so that they are maximum with peak concentrations of levodopa, are accentuated at the start and end of each dose, or are most marked in the early morning. Close observation of the individual patient and, where appropriate, administration of smaller but more frequent doses may be useful. Since dyskinesias relate to the effect of levodopa on the corpus striatum, the concomitant administration of decarboxylase inhibitors has no effect on their incidence.

Prolonged treatment with levodopa often is accompanied by complex response patterns in which there are swings from relative mobility to periods of profound akinesia. These usually occur as the disease becomes more and more resistant to levodopa, so that instead of being effective for 3–6 h, each dose produces improvement only for 1–2 h. Occasionally the cycles are much more frequent, so that up to ten cycles of mobility and akinesia may occur within half an hour. One approach is to give smaller doses of levodopa more frequently. This works where changes in performance relate to changes in drug blood levels. If this is not the cause, modification of dosage is unlikely to have much effect. Many authorities consider that the "on-off" pattern is the result of levodopa prolonging the lives of patients to a late stage of Parkinson's disease rather than a consequence of prolonged therapy.

Amantadine

This is an antiviral agent which has an unexplained effect on dopamine receptors in Parkinson's disease. It may be used in synergy with levodopa. It causes restlessness, nervousness, and irritability in a fifth of patients and visual hallucinations in up to a tenth. Mottling of the skin (livedo reticularis) also may occur. These side-effects and the fact that its benefit rarely is sustained for more than 6 months mean that it now has only a small role in the treatment of Parkinson's disease. In old people it merely complicates a drug regime without conferring much real benefit.

Bromocriptine

Amongst other activities the ergot derivative bromocriptine has been found to be effective in the treatment of Parkinson's disease. Its main mode of action in this respect is that it is a dopamine agonist which stimulates postsynaptic dopamine receptors in the corpus striatum. Like levodopa it is effective in reducing akinesia, rigidity, and tremor in Parkinsonism. An important difference from levodopa is that it has a longer duration of action, having a half-life of 6–8 h. It is much easier therefore to achieve steady blood concentrations.

The drug can cause nausea, but this occurs much less commonly than with levodopa. Postural changes in blood pressure are of the same order as those with levodopa. Other vascular effects include Raynaud's phenomenon and redness and mild oedema of the arms and legs. Dyskinetic movements occur if too large a dose is given but are no more troublesome than with levodopa.

Much more on the debit side is that it often causes agitation and confusion and, more specifically, vivid visual hallucinations and convincing paranoid delusions. These problems are particularly common in old age and occur with bromocriptine with far greater frequency than with levodopa. They also often persist for several weeks after treatment is discontinued.

Bromocriptine, then, is as effective in Parkinson's disease as levodopa, but its serious psychiatric side-effects and high cost limit its use to special circumstances. An example is that it can be given to patients in whom levodopa causes nausea and vomiting. Again, in the later stages of Parkinson's disease its more constant blood levels are useful in the patient exhibiting major swings in function while on levodopa. It also can be tried with benefit in a patient whose disease is becoming increasingly refractory to levodopa. Patients who show a poor initial response to levodopa, however, usually do not do any better on bromocriptine.

More recently it has become clear that side-effects often were due to starting on too large a dose of the drug. It may be that if smaller doses are used the drug will prove to be a more acceptable alternative to levodopa in the initial treatment of Parkinsonism.

The effective dose varies a lot, but commonly lies between 10 and 30 mg three times daily. Side-effects are best minimised by starting on 2.5 mg daily and only increasing this by 2.5 mg every alternate day. If it is used in conjunction with levodopa, 3.5–10 mg should be considered to be the equivalent of 100 mg of the latter. This is only an approximation, however, and a much greater variation in dosage may be necessary.

Other Extrapyramidal Disorders

Orofacial Dyskinesia

Writhing movements of the lips and tongue are found characteristically in patients receiving long-term psychiatric care. The abnormality here is due to the administration of massive doses of phenothiazines. Elderly patients with mental impairment may be on phenothiazines, but few are on large enough doses to cause dyskinesia. A more common cause in this group is levodopa overdosage. Treatment consists of reducing the dose of the offending drug.

There remains a small group of old people in whom dyskinesia is the result, not of drugs, but of gliosis in the midbrain and substantia nigra. This form may respond to tetrabenazine, a drug which produces catecholamine depletion of the corpus striatum. Dosage is 25 mg three times daily, increasing this to a maximum of 200 mg daily. Catecholamine imbalance also may be modified by using a phenothiazine such as thioproprazate hydrochloride. Since old people are particularly sensitive to these drugs they should be used with extreme caution. In fact, if the dyskinesia is not particularly distressing it may be best left untreated.

Chorea

Chorea is a condition characterised by continuous random jerking movements of the face and limbs. A wide range of abnormalities may be responsible (Table 10.3). In senile chorea there are degenerative changes in the corpus striatum, while in unilateral chorea there usually is infarction of the contralateral subthalamic nucleus.

Table 10.3. Causes of chorea in the elderly (the more common are italicised)

Generalised chorea	*Chorea due to drugs*
Sydenham's chorea	Huntington's chorea
Chorea in thyrotoxicosis	*Senile chorea*
Chorea in systemic lupus erythematosus	Sydenham's chorea
Chorea in polycythaemia	*Stroke*
Chorea in encephalitis lethargica	Tumour
Chorea in osteomalacia	Thalamotomy
Chorea in hepatic cirrhosis	

Pharmacological intervention in senile or vascular chorea aims at correcting the relative excess of dopamine over acetylcholine found in brain tissues of affected individuals. Table 10.4 lists some of these approaches. The only ones of proven value are those of thioproprazate and tetrabenazine. Since tetrabenazine has few side-effects it is the drug of first choice, thioproprazate being reserved for patients failing to respond to this. In theory the alcohol dimethylaminoethanol (deanol) should work, in that it delivers high concentrations of the acetylcholine substrate choline to the corpus striatum. Unfortunately there have been no controlled trials of efficacy in senile chorea.

Table 10.4. Pharmacological management of choreiform movement disorders

Mechanism	Drugs
1. Blockage of dopamine receptors	Thioproprazate hydrochloride
2. Dopamine depletion	Tetrabenazine
3. Reduced receptor sensitivity to dopamine	Lithium carbonate
4. Increased acetylcholine levels	Physostigmine
	Deanol

Hemiballismus

This consists of violent flinging or rotational movements of the arm. It usually is related to infarction of the contralateral subthalamic nucleus. The recommended treatment is to give the phenothiazine perphenazine in a dose of 6–24 mg/day. There must be the usual caveat that old people have increased sensitivity to phenothiazines, so they should be started on a minimal dose, which should be increased only if there are no disabling side-effects. In view of this problem there is the need for a careful evaluation of other forms of therapy, such as tetrabenazine, in the condition.

Tremor

Essential tremor is a benign condition presenting as a coarse tremor unrelated to movement and not associated with other neurological abnormalities. Though it may occur at any age it is particularly common in the elderly. A large proportion of subjects respond to the administration of propranolol. Unfortunately, the degree of response bears an inverse relationship to the age of the patient, but even in extreme old age it is well worth trying. The recommended dosage is 40 mg propranolol three times daily, but in the elderly an impaired first-pass metabolism usually indicates a much smaller starting dose, say, 10 mg three times per day (Chap. 1).

The tremor also may be controlled by diazepam, but the drug's serious sedative effects and long half-life limit its usefulness in old age. It has long been recognised that the tremor may be abolished by a stiff drink of alcohol. In view of a rising incidence of alcoholism even in the elderly, patients should be discouraged from turning to this as a remedy.

Epilepsy

Epilepsy is common in patients admitted to a geriatric unit (Table 10.5). The most common cause is cerebrovascular disease, but other causes such as a meningioma, hypoglycaemia, or cardiac arrhythmia should be excluded. Where the condition persists a wide range of drugs are available (Table 10.6).

The choice of drug is governed primarily by the type of epilepsy, in that treatment of petit mal seizures differs from that of grand mal ones. Many old

Table 10.5. Causes of epilepsy in the elderly (Hildick-Smith 1974)

Cerebrovascular and/or dementia	28
Cerebral tumour	5
Metabolic	4
"Idiopathic" (epilepsy from childhood)	4
Intermittent heart block	1
Post-traumatic	1
Unknown cause	7
Total	50

Table 10.6. Drugs used in the treatment of epilepsy

Type of epilepsy	Drug
Petit mal	Ethosuximide (with phenytoin or phenobarbitone) Clonazepam Sodium valproate
Grand mal and partial seisure	*First-line drugs* Phenytoin Carbamazepine Phenobarbitone and congeners *Second-line drugs* Clonazepam Sodium valproate Sulthiame

people suffer from focal forms of epilepsy, which may present with a wide range of symptoms including confusion, pain, or hallucinations. Drug treatment for these is the same as for grand mal seizures. Consideration should also be given to the duration of action of drugs. Phenytoin and particularly phenobarbitone have long half-lives, so that they need only be given once daily to old people. Carbamazepine with a half-life of only 12 h may have to be given twice daily. A long half-life has the advantage of improving compliance, but the disadvantage of delaying the disappearance of side-effects if the drug has to be withdrawn.

Toxicity also influences choice of drugs used in grand mal epilepsy (Table 10.7). Phenobarbitone is the one most likely to cause severe drowsiness, while phenytoin is most likely to cause ataxia and diplopia. Phenytoin is the only one to cause gum hypertrophy and hirsutism, but this rarely is a serious problem in old age. Folic acid and vitamin D depletion are due to anticonvulsants inducing their metabolism by liver enzymes, but should not create difficulty if haemoglobin and calcium and alkaline phosphatase concentrations are checked regularly. Carbamazepine has been reported as causing marrow aplasia, but this probably happens no more frequently than with many other drugs. In terms of overall side-effects, phenytoin is marginally less toxic in old people than phenobarbitone. Carbamazepine is not nearly so widely used in old people as phenobarbitone or phenytoin, probably because it is a newer drug and slightly more expensive.

Table 10.7 Side-effects of phenobarbitone, phenytoin, and carbamazepine

Side-effect	Phenobarbitone	Phenytoin	Carbamazepine
Drowsiness	+ + +	+	+ +
Cerebellar and ocular muscle dysfunction	+ +	+	+
Gum hypertrophy	−	+	−
Hirsutism	−	+	−
Folic acid depletion	+	+	+
Vitamin D depletion	+	+	−
Rashes	+	+	+
Blood dyscrasia	±	±	±

+ + + Very common; + + Common; + Occasional; ± Rare.

In achieving a maximum therapeutic effect and avoiding side-effects, information on the blood concentration of an anticonvulsant is critical. The optimal range for phenobarbitone is 15–40 μg/ml, for phenytoin 10–20 μg/ml, and for carbamazepine 4–10 μg/ml (Reynolds 1978). The relationship between the dose of phenytoin and blood concentrations is such that there is a critical dosage above which the hepatic enzyme system is saturated and there is a much steeper rise of blood concentrations. Ageing impairs phenytoin metabolism, and the optimal dose usually is about 300 mg/day. The long half-life of phenytoin means that 5–10 days are required to achieve a steady concentration. There is therefore little point in checking the serum phenytoin concentration much before 2 weeks after the start of medication. If, at this stage, the concentration is suboptimal, dosage should be increased from 300 to 350 or 400 mg daily, depending upon the value of the concentration. If, despite this, the concentration still remains suboptimal, dosage should be increased further, but in view of the saturation kinetics of phenytoin, single increments of more than 100 mg should be avoided. It might be argued that the routine measurement of plasma anticonvulsant concentrations could be replaced by careful clinical observation, but there is convincing evidence that monitoring these improves anticonvulsant control.

There have been no recent studies on the kinetics of phenobarbitone or carbamazepine in elderly epileptics. This is particularly unfortunate in the case of carbamazepine because of its shorter half-life. Again, the linear relationship between dosage and blood concentrations would make it an easier drug to use than phenytoin. At present, in the elderly, carbamazepine should probably be started at 200 mg daily, increasing by 100 mg every week until effective blood concentrations have been reached.

In many patients, optimal plasma concentrations of anticonvulsants may not have to be maintained to control seizures. If therefore a patient is troubled by side-effects, such as drowsiness or ataxia, it may be worth cautiously reducing dosage rather than switching to another anticonvulsant.

If convulsions are not being controlled there is a strong temptation to add a second or even a third anticonvulsant. This has considerable disadvantages. First, it complicates treatment making compliance less likely. Again, there may be unpredictable interactions. Phenobarbitone, for example, may either increase or decrease plasma concentrations of phenytoin (Table 10.8). Anticonvulsant activity may also be modified by a wide range of other agents, and vice versa (Table 10.8).

Before adding another anticonvulsant, then, the first step is to ensure that optimal plasma concentrations of the first one have been reached. If this does not provide seizure control, another drug should be introduced, gradually reducing the dosage of the first, until the second one has replaced it. Only if this fails should two drugs be used together.

Old people may present in status epilepticus. Here, as in any age group, treatment consists of slow intravenous infusion of either diazepam or clonazepam. In the elderly, even greater care should be taken to monitor for respiratory or cardiovascular depression.

Table 10.8. Anticonvulsants and drug interactions

Drug	Drug causing interaction	Mechanism of interaction	Effect of interaction
Phenytoin	Phenobarbitone	Saturation of enzymes Enzyme induction	Raised phenytoin level Reduced phenytoin level
Phenytoin	Sodium valproate	Displacement from plasma protein	Increased phenytoin activity
Phenytoin	Carbamazepine	Enzyme induction	Reduced phenytoin level
Phenytoin	Isoniazid	Inhibition of metabolism	Increased phenytoin level
Phenytoin	Phenylbutazone	Displacement of plasma protein	Increased phenytoin level
Phenytoin	Alcohol	Enzyme induction	Reduced phenytoin level
Corticosteroids	Phenobarbitone Phenytoin	Enzyme induction	Reduced steroid level
Vitamin D Folic acid	Phenobarbitone Phenytoin	Enzyme induction	Reduced vitamin D and folate levels

NB: This table is not comprehensive.

Peripheral Nerve Disorders

Herpes Zoster

An infection with herpes zoster can have a devastating effect on an elderly patient, converting a healthy and cheerful individual into a depressed and housebound cripple. An important factor in this is the high incidence of postherpetic neuralgia. A large range of analgesics and local applications have been tried but all found wanting. The most effective approach is to treat the active lesion with the antiviral agent idoxuridine. This is prepared as a 5% solution in dimethylsulphoxide, a solvent which is absorbed transcutaneously. If the drug is to be effective it should be applied as soon as the infection develops, preferably before the eruption of vesicles. Applications should be repeated four times a day for 4 days or until the rash has subsided.

Antiviral agents have been used systemically in herpes encephalitis. This is confined mainly to patients on immunosuppressive therapy and rarely occurs in otherwise healthy old people.

Trigeminal Neuralgia

This is another painful peripheral nerve lesion which is particularly common in old age. The mainstay of drug treatment here is carbamazepine. This produces immediate pain relief in 70% of patients. During exacerbations of neuralgia 100 mg carbamazepine may have to be taken up to three-hourly. Maintenance dosage ranges between 100 and 200 mg twice daily. Those not controlled by carbamazepine usually benefit from surgery such as local alcohol injection.

Special Senses

Hearing

While drugs rarely improve hearing, there are a wide range of them which may impair it. Old people are particularly susceptible in that they already may have substantial hearing loss, and poor renal function exacerbates the effects of ototoxic substances. Gentamycin causes deafness by destroying hair cells within the cochlea and vestibule. Vestibular damage often is more extensive than that to the cochlea, so that a disturbed balance may be more prominent than hearing loss. Damage can be minimised if blood gentamycin levels are kept to between 4 and 6 μg/ml 2 h after an injection, and below 2 μg/ml before the next injection. Even a marginal increase of gentamycin levels over the therapeutic range may be enough to cause severe damage, in that the endolymph tends to concentrate aminoglycosides to levels well in excess of those in the plasma. These levels may be maintained for long after the drug has been withdrawn. Patients should thus be followed up for several weeks to ensure that there has been no ototoxicity.
    Streptomycin also may be responsible for serious labyrinthine disorders. The risk is reduced if dosage in the elderly is limited to 500 mg/day. At present the use of streptomycin has been reduced by replacing it and para-aminosalicylic acid in routine antituberculous therapy with ethambutol and rifampicin (Chap. 5).
    Loop diuretics such as frusemide and particularly ethacrynic acid have a direct toxic effect on hair cell receptors of the cochlea and labyrinth. Usually the hearing disturbance is temporary, but if aminoglycosides also are being given the ototoxic effects of the latter are potentiated. The type of clinical situation in which this might occur would be a patient with subacute bacterial endocarditis due to *Streptococcus faecalis* who also was in cardiac failure.
    Salicylates also may be responsible for hearing loss and tinnitus. These changes always are temporary and disappear when the drug is stopped. Reports of permanent hearing loss due to salicylates have not been substantiated.

Balance

Attacks of dizziness are a common cause of falls in old people, and result in a great deal of anxiety amongst relatives and social work and health care professionals. The attacks may be described as dizziness rather than vertigo because old people give a rather vague account of them and fail to give a classical description of vertigo. Treatment is dependent on the cause. This may be postural hypotension or a transient arrhythmia (Chap. 4). Drugs such as phenothiazines, anticonvulsants, and antidepressants may be responsible, and stopping them often resolves the problem. In other patients there is ischaemia of vestibular nuclei, and treatment of hypertension may control this. Vestibular sedatives such as prochlorperazine may work, but, by suppressing peripheral reflexes, they often make any imbalance worse.

A history of deafness combined with dizziness is suggestive of peripheral vestibular damage. This can be treated with an antihistamine such as cinnarizine 15–30 mg three times daily or dimenhydrinate 50 mg three times a day. Surprisingly, patients also respond well to betahistine 8 mg eight-hourly. This is a histamine agonist with a vasodilator effect. The suggestion is that whereas antihistamines act as vestibular sedatives, betahistine improves the blood supply to the labyrinth.

Sometimes patients with labyrinthine disease do not present with dizziness or vertigo. An example is that many old people describing classical drop attacks, on testing, have evidence of labyrinthine disease and respond well to cinnarizine.

Vision

Certain diseases of the eye which are particularly common in old people show an effective response to drugs. An example is ocular herpes zoster, whose management has been revolutionised by the development of idoxuridine. This is available as 0.1% eye drops or a 0.5% eye ointment. An important caveat is that 5% idoxuridine in dimethyl sulphoxide is highly irritant to mucosal surfaces and should *never* be applied to the eye.

Another condition responding to medication is primary open-angle glaucoma. Its incidence increases with age (Fig. 10.4). Parasympatheticomimetic drugs such as pilocarpine or physostigmine improve the flow of aqueous humour to the canal of Schlem by contracting the iris. The carbonic anhydrase inhibitor acetazolamide, when taken orally, reduces the flow of bicarobonate and, as a consequence, water into the aqueous fluid. Finally, beta-blocking agents also are effective in reducing the formation of aqueous humour. The one of choice is timolol maleate prepared as 0.25% or 0.5% drops.

Drugs which block the canal of Schlem by widening the iris may cause a rise in the intra-ocular pressure. Culprits include drugs with anticholinergic effect, such as the phenothiazine tranquillisers, tricyclic antidepressants, and urinary bladder relaxants. The side-effect usually is a theoretical rather than a practical problem. It is enough merely to be on the alert for a deterioration in vision in

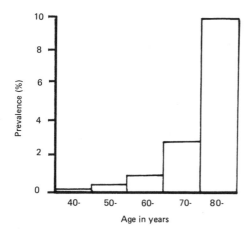

Fig. 10.4. Prevalence of primary open-angle glaucoma related to age (Crick 1980).

patients on these drugs and to avoid their use in patients with a history of glaucoma.

References

Acheson J, Danta G, Hutchinson EC (1969) Controlled trial of dipyridamole in cerebral vascular disease. Br Med J 1: 614–615

Admani AK (1978) New approach to treatment of recent stroke. Br Med J 2: 1678–1679

Calne DB, Stern GM, Spiers ASD, Lawrence DR, Armitage P (1969) L-dopa in idiopathic Parkinsonism. Lancet 2: 973–976

Canadian Cooperative Study Group (1978) A randomised trial of aspirin and sulphinpyrazone in threatened stroke. New Engl J Med 299: 54–59

Crick RP (1980) Glaucoma—the present situation. Practitioner 224: 621–632

Fields WS (1979) Role of antiplatelet agents in cerebrovascular disease. Drugs 18: 150–155

Hildick-Smith M (1974) Epilepsy in the elderly. Age Ageing 3: 203–208

Kannel WB, Wolf P, Dawber TR (1978) Hypertension and cardiac impairments increase stroke risk. Geriatrics 33: 71–83

Marshall J (1976) The management of cerebrovascular disease. Churchill Livingstone, London

Millikan CH (1979) Anticoagulant therapy for prevention of stroke. Med Clin North Am 63: 897–904

Mitchell JRA (1979) Does aspirin prevent stroke? Practitioner 223: 668–674

Parkes JD (1981) Adverse effects of antiparkinsonian drugs. Drugs 21: 341–353

Reynolds EH (1978) Drug treatment of epilepsy. Lancet 2: 721–725

Shaw KM, Lees AJ, Stern GM (1980) The impact of treatment with levodopa on Parkinson's disease. Q J Med 49: 283–293

White NJ, Barnes TRE (1981) Senile Parkinsonism, a survey of current treatment. Age Ageing 10: 105–109

11 Mental Disorders

Insomnia

Young people usually find sleep easily. As they age, sleep becomes increasingly fragmented and less and less deep. The normal sleep pattern deteriorates with increasing age to such an extent that it is often of an erratic pattern characterised by frequent "cat-naps" rather than being sustained.

Periods of wakefulness are a natural concomitant of increasing age and should not necessarily be considered as requiring a hypnotic in preference to patient reassurance. Reasonable diagnostic efforts should be made before hypnotic drugs are prescribed, and obvious factors involved in the aetiology of insomnia must be considered, for example, nocturnal pain and discomfort (e.g. peptic ulcer, nocturnal angina, and arthritic pain). Caffeine, alcohol, noise, and drugs all contribute to insomnia. All possible steps must be taken to remove these causes before considering the administration of a hypnotic.

Hypnotics

The most commonly prescribed hypnotics are the benzodiazepines. As a group they are thought to have advantages over other agents in terms of a greater safety margin, fewer side-effects, and a lower potential of serious interactions with other drugs. This, in turn, has led to their extensive use in the elderly.

In spite of their excellent safety record and apparent advantages over other hypnotics such as the barbiturates, benzodiazepines have the disadvantages inherent in any drug which acts by suppressing the central nervous system. These disadvantages are particularly evident in old age.

The frequency of drowsiness, mental impairment, and ataxia associated with diazepam, chlordiazepoxide, flurazepam, and nitrazepam increases steadily with age. Their severity is clearly related to the dosage used. Thus, though they occur when doses appropriate to younger individuals are used, they often disappear when lower but effective doses are prescribed.

It was originally thought that the explanation for the increase in adverse drug reactions might be a change in drug pharmacokinetics. However, it is now established that the elderly make significantly more mistakes in psychomotor testing then young controls, even though both groups have similar plasma concentrations and half-lives of the benzodiazepines. This suggests that there is a direct increase in the sensitivity of the ageing brain to benzodiazepines. This probably is due to an age-related reduction in the number of benzodiazepine receptors, so that a greater proportion of those surviving are occupied by benzodiazepines.

This increased sensitivity to the benzodiazepines in the elderly undoubtedly accounts in part for the increased frequency of unwanted central effects observed in many controlled drug studies. If treatment with hypnotics is required, then benzodiazepines should be prescribed in doses lower than those required for young healthy adults (Table 11.1). In addition to prescribing lower dosages, there is a suggestion that the shorter-acting benzodiazepines may be freer of side-effects than those which are longer-acting, but the evidence for this is as yet inconclusive.

Table 11.1. Suggested doses of hypnotics for use in the elderly

Drug	Dose
Nitrazepam	2.5–5 mg
Temazepam	5 20 mg
Chlormethiazole	250–500 mg
Triclofos	0.5–1.0 g

Barbiturates should not be used as hypnotics in the elderly or, indeed, in any age group, as there is a high incidence of side-effects and they are dangerous in overdosage.

Occasionally doctors encounter patients who have been on barbiturate hypnotics for many years. If the patient is well there is no problem, but if he is drowsy, confused, or ataxic an attempt should be made to change therapy. The best way of doing this is gradually to reduce the dose of the barbiturate, replacing it with a gradually increasing dose of a short-acting benzodiazepine. The best solution would be to withdraw hypnotic therapy altogether, but this is extremely difficult in a patient who has been on treatment for years.

Triclofos and chlormethiazole have the advantage over the benzodiazepines that they are currently available in syrup form. Chlormethiazole is as effective a hypnotic as temazepam and has been reported to cause less confusion than other hypnotics in the elderly. It is, however, less safe than the benzodiazepines in that it is more likely to cause death after accidental over-dosage. Despite this, it is a useful hypnotic in the confused elderly patient.

In summary, if the need has been established, an elderly patient should be prescribed a short course of hypnotics to "normalise" the sleep pattern, taking care to use a safe preparation, preferably with a short duration of action and in a lower dosage than that required for healthy young adults.

Depression

Depressive illness is common in the elderly and continues to rise with increasing age. In the case of recurrent depressive illness, there is an increase in the frequency of attacks.

Depression may result from many causes, e.g. severe illness or the death of a spouse, moving away of children, retirement, moving home, and probably most important, acute physical illness, particularly a stroke. Depression in the older age group is frequently difficult to diagnose in the early stages, often presenting as sleep, memory, or concentration disturbances, lack of drive, or somatic symptoms. It is particularly important, in this respect, to distinguish between dementia and the "pseudodementia" of depression.

Traditionally psychiatrists thought that depression occurring for the first time in later life was a forerunner of dementia. Whilst it has been shown that many patients with depression do develop multi-infarct or senile dementia, these do not occur more frequently than would be expected in an age-matched sample of the general population. Therefore, although depression is more common in the elderly and depressive symptoms more common in dementia, the two conditions are entirely separate entities.

Often it is difficult to differentiate between depression and organic disease and it is necessary for a very careful history and examination with particular attention to concurrent drug therapy to be undertaken before making a diagnosis of depression.

Many drugs commonly prescribed for the elderly have been associated with depression. These include antihypertensive agents (reserpine, methyldopa, hydralazine, clonidine, and propranolol), anti-Parkinsonian agents (levodopa, bromocriptine, and amantadine), hormones (oestrogen and progesterone), and corticosteroids.

Tricyclic Antidepressants

This group contains both the most effective and largest number of compounds used in the treatment of depression. The main mode of action is thought to be a block of neuronal re-uptake of amines in the central nervous system, thus potentiating their central actions.

There is no doubt that the tricyclics are effective antidepressants in the young and old alike. The elderly are, however, more susceptible to the anticholinergic and anti-alpha-adrenergic side-effects, particularly urinary retention, constipation, postural hypotension, blurred vision, and confusion. Therefore, like most centrally acting drugs used in the elderly, care must be taken in their administration, preferably starting with small doses and increasing gradually until an effective therapeutic dose has been achieved. It may take a considerable time to arrive at the optimal dose, since a therapeutic response may be delayed by 10 days or more from commencement of therapy. Problems of compliance are reduced by giving an antidepressant as a single evening dose.

Since polypharmacy is common in the elderly, particular care should be taken to avoid the wide range of interactions associated with tricyclic agents (Table 11.2).

Table 11.2. Interactions with tricyclic antidepressants

Drugs	Nature of interaction
Sedatives, hypnotics, and alcohol	Increased sedation with the sedative tricyclics
Anti-Parkinsonian drugs and phenothiazines	Increased anticholinergic effects
Antihypertensive drugs	Increased postural hypotension
Clonidine	Antagonism of antihypertensive effect
Monoamine oxidase inhibitors	Hypertension, excitement, hyperpyrexia, and convulsions

Patients with cardiac disease, particularly with associated arrhythmias, are particularly at risk from the tricyclics and therefore great care must be exercised in their prescription.

The choice of tricyclic depends on the nature of the presentation of the depression. If there is serious sleep disturbance a tricyclic with a sedative effect should be prescribed. Examples include amitriptyline and dothiepin (Table 11.3).

Table 11.3. Sedative effects of tricyclic antidepressants

No sedation	Protriptyline
Mild sedation	Desipramine, nortriptyline
Moderate sedation	Imipramine, dothiepin
Most sedative	Trimipramine, amitriptyline, doxepin
Least likely to produce cardiac arrhythmias	Doxepin

Monoamine Oxidase Inhibitors

This group of drugs is generally less effective and more hazardous than the tricyclics in the treatment of depression. Their mode of action is to increase the brain content of monoamines by inhibiting monoamine oxidase activity. This, in turn, leads to a potentiation of central noradrenergic function and an improvement in the patient's mood and symptoms. Like the tricyclics their effect may be delayed by several weeks from commencement of therapy.

Their use is contraindicated in patients with epilepsy or severe liver disease and in those unlikely to observe dietary restrictions, where there is a risk of precipitating fits, encephalopathy, and hypertensive crisis. The elderly patient is more at risk primarily owing to poor dietary compliance.

Anticholinergic effects are common, particularly with the higher doses, and a hypertensive crisis often follows the ingestion of tyramine- or dopamine-containing foods such as Bovril or Marmite and some beers and common cold remedies. Therefore, great care must be exercised in their prescription and dietary advice must be carefully outlined to all patients receiving this group of drugs (Table 11.4). Any suggestion of confusion in an elderly patient should be acted upon and, if necessary, the drug withdrawn. For these reasons, mono-amine oxidase inhibitors should only be used in patients in whom treatment with the tricyclic antidepressants has failed, and should only be prescribed after a psychiatric consultation.

Table 11.4. Drug interactions with monoamine oxidase inhibitors

Foods containing tyramine or dopamine, e.g. Bovril, Marmite
Indirect sympatheticomimetic amines, e.g. ephedrine, phenyl
  propranolamine (common cold remedies)
Tricyclic and tetracyclic antidepressants
Pethidine (and other narcotics)
Reserpine and tetrabenazine
Anticholinergics
Insulin and hypoglycaemic drugs
Antihypertensive drugs

Lithium Carbonate

Lithium carbonate was first introduced as a treatment of mania in 1949 and now has established itself as part of the management of manic depressive psychoses. In controlled studies it is not generally an effective treatment of acute endogenous depression nor of schizophrenia, but has been shown to be superior to imipramine and placebo as a maintenance therapy in manic depressive disorders. Its mode of action is unclear, but its effect of increasing the intracellular sodium concentration by interference with the sodium/potassium ionic pump may be important.

Lithium carbonate has a narrow therapeutic window and care must therefore be exercised in its use because of its toxic side-effects. Renal impairment and dehydration as a result of diarrhoea, vomiting, or diuretic therapy cause accumulation of lithium and this predisposes to toxicity. In addition, a reduced creatinine clearance means that the elderly usually need smaller doses to maintain satisfactory plasma levels and therapeutic efficacy.

The use of lithium carbonate predisposes to hypothyroidism (and goitre) so that six-monthly checks of thyroid function are necessary. Other signs of toxicity include vomiting and severe diarrhoea, muscle twitching, drowsiness, dysarthria and vertigo with tremor, and weight gain. Oedema and thirst with polyuria often occur even at therapeutic levels. As in the case of monoamine oxidase inhibitors, treatment should probably only be initiated on the advice of a psychiatrist.

Tetracyclic and Other Antidepressant Drugs

Mianserin and, to a lesser extent, maprotiline currently have many advocates in the treatment of depression in the elderly. The reason for their increase in use has been the suggestion that they are safer in accidental overdosage and have fewer anticholinergic side-effects than tricyclics. This may result from their rather more selective inhibition of 5-hydroxytryptamine uptake into the adrenergic neurone. Despite this, reactions and side-effects of tetracyclics are broadly similar to those of tricyclic antidepressants, with drowsiness occurring more commonly, particularly when they are given along with hypnotic sedatives or alcohol. Again, though experience varies and comparative trials are difficult to interpret, many psychiatrists feel that they are less effective than tricyclic agents and continue to use the latter as their first choice. They reserve tetracyclics for patients in whom tricyclics produce intolerable side-effects.

Dosage, as with other antidepressants and centrally acting drugs, must be tailored to the need of the individual, starting at lower dosages and gradually increasing until a therapeutic effect is noted. The associated drowsiness with the initial therapy of mianserin appears to decrease after several days administration, but is often troublesome in the early stages.

Confusion

Confusion is a symptom common in the elderly. It is usually associated with underlying organic disease. It also may occur as a direct result of medication prescribed for other conditions.

The list of therapeutic agents capable of producing confusion in the elderly is extremely long (Table 11.5). Drug-induced confusion can result from decreased metabolism, reduced renal or hepatic function, or increased sensitivity of the central nervous system to the drugs. No drug cures confusion. Cures only come from treatment of the underlying cause where it can be detected, for example, infection or drug therapy.

An accurate diagnosis is essential in the management of confusion and depends on a good clinical history and examination. This, combined with expert

Table 11.5. Causes of confusion in the elderly

Infection	Pneumonia
	Urinary tract infection
	Meningitis
Drugs	Digoxin, reserpine, methyldopa, sedatives, alcohol,
	anticholinergics, anti-Parkinsonians, tricyclic
	antidepressants, anxiolytics, antipsychotics, cimetidine
Organic brain disease	Cerebral infarction
	Haematoma or tumour
	Alzheimer's disease
Metabolic and endocrine	Thyroid disease
	Diabetes mellitus
	Dehydration
	Electrolyte disturbance
	Hepatic or renal failure
Nutritional	Anaemia (B_{12} and iron deficiency)
	Vitamin deficiencies
Miscellaneous	Depression
	Situational change
	Hypothermia

nursing with an emphasis on hydration and early mobilisation, can improve most patients' confusional states. If an organic cause for the confusion cannot be identified or if treatment of the disorder has not produced a rapid improvement, a major tranquilliser may have to be prescribed. The choice of tranquilliser is usually an individual one based upon prejudices and previous experience.

All major tranquillisers act by blocking dopamine receptors in the basal ganglia and limbic areas, with the result that many of their side-effects are related to this same action. Side-effects which are particularly troublesome in the elderly are sedation, agitation, increased confusion, Parkinsonism (extrapyramidal), akathesia and dystonic reactions, tardive dyskinesia (often irreversible), postural hypotension (anti-adrenergic), constipation and urinary retention (anticholinergic), and hypothermia.

The three main classes of major tranquillisers are the phenothiazines, thioxanthines, and butyrophenones. All cause extrapyramidal effects and sedation, and their prescribed dose must be tailored to produce maximal efficacy with minimal side-effects. In general the elderly are more susceptible to the side-effects of these drugs and special care must be used in patients who have hepatic or renal impairment. Treatment should start at lower doses, for example, thioridazine 10–12.5 mg three times daily, promazine and chlorpromazine 25 mg daily, or haloperidol 0.5–1.5 mg three times daily. Haloperidol is very useful in controlling the very agitated patient and can be given intramuscularly if required in a dosage of 5–10 mg.

Many patients benefit from a single evening dose, say, 50 mg thioridazine or 100 mg chlorpromazine. This controls nocturnal restlessness and often provides sufficient sedation during the next day to provide control without producing excessive drowsiness.

Chronic Mental Impairment

The attention which medieval alchemists devoted towards finding an elixir of youth is now lavished on finding an effective treatment for senile and multi-infarct dementias. It could be argued that the theoretical basis for the use of many preparations recommended in this field is ill-founded and that their clinical efficacy is, to say the least, unproven. The people who appear to have benefited most appear to have been doctors who have obtained research publications and pharmaceutical companies who have managed to develop large markets for many of the agents. This, however, is an unfair judgement. In the United Kingdom alone there are around 150 000 old people with severe dementia who exact a high financial, physical, and emotional cost from their families and from the community in general. A search for effective treatment thus is not only justified but, in a world with a rapidly ageing population, is a matter of extreme urgency. When investigations are performed in this field, however, it is important that certain basic principles be observed.

Diagnosis

The first principle is that the dementia under investigation should be defined accurately. It may be that mental impairment is the wrong diagnosis. Old people with deafness, dysarthria, dysphasia, or akinesia all too often are labelled as being "senile". Again, apathy, unresponsiveness, and self-neglect may be the result of depression rather than dementia. Once these conditions have been excluded, it has to be recognised that people with mental impairment form a heterogeneous group suffering from a wide range of different disorders (Table 11.6). In some instances, early identification and treatment should restore mental function almost to normal. Examples include the evacuation of a subdural haemorrhage, removal of a meningioma or drainage of a normal-pressure hydrocephalus. In others treatment will at least halt further deterioration. Examples include thyroxine in hypothyroidism, hydroxycobalamin in B_{12} deficiency, or penicillin in neurosyphilis. In the remainder, an accurate diagnosis at least makes it possible to ensure that a drug under scrutiny is being used in a homogeneous population.

Although careful investigation may turn up a wide range of disorders in demented elderly patients, the clinician finds that, at the end of the day, most of his patients suffer from either Alzheimer's disease or multi-infarct dementia. In terms of general management the distinction between these two disorders does not matter greatly. If, however, a drug with a well-defined mode of action is

Table 11.6. Causes of mental impairment in the elderly

Alzheimer's disease	*Subnutrition*
Multiple cerebral infarcts	B_{12} deficiency
	Folic acid deficiency
Trauma	Nicotinic acid deficiency
Subdural haemorrhage	Potassium deficiency
Multiple injuries (e.g. boxing)	
	Infection
Tumours	Neurosyphilis
Meningioma	Chronic pyelonephritis
Primary malignant cerebral tumour	
Secondary cerebral tumour	*Cardiorespiratory*
Carcinomatous encephalopathy	Anoxia
	Hypercapnia
Normal-pressure hydrocephalus	
	Drugs
Metabolic and endocrine	Tranquillisers
Hypothyroidism	Sedatives
Thyrotoxicosis	Hypnotics
Hypercalcaemia (e.g. hyperparathyroidism, vitamin D	Anti-Parkinsonians
intoxication, multiple myeloma)	Diuretics
Hyponatraemia (e.g. diuretics, gastro-intestinal upset,	Cardiac glycosides
inappropriate ADH secretion)	
Hypokalaemia (e.g. diuretics, subnutrition)	
Hypoglycaemia (e.g. insulinoma, treatment of diabetes)	
Uraemia (e.g. dehydration, chronic renal failure)	
Chronic liver disease	

under scrutiny the distinction may matter a great deal. Alzheimer's disease is due to neuronal dysfunction associated with specific neurotransmitter deficiencies, whereas multi-infarct dementia is the result of neuronal destruction or dysfunction due to cerebral anoxia. A drug designed to improve cerebral circulation might not be expected to work in Alzheimer's disease, whilst one replacing neurotransmitters would not work in multi-infarct dementia.

Unfortunately, it can be difficult to make the distinction between the two disorders on a clinical basis. Lloyd-Evans et al. (1978) devised a scoring system for arteriosclerosis, but found that they obtained a similar range of scores in demented and non-demented subjects. They concluded, therefore, that the test merely identified patients with coincidental dementia and arteriosclerosis, but failed to distinguish between patients with Alzheimer's disease and multi-infarct dementia.

Isaacs (1979) proposed that in identifying a group of patients with Alzheimer's disease, those subjects should be excluded who have a previous history of cerebrovascular disease; who have had a myocardial infarction; who have evidence of peripheral vascular disease; who have a diastolic pressure over 100 mm Hg, an ESR over 50 mm/1st hour, or a haemoglobin of less than 11 g/dl;

who have disease of the cardiovascular, renal, hepatic, or endocrine systems; who have evidence of renal or respiratory infection or evidence of cancer; or who are receiving drugs.

For these criteria to receive wide acceptance it would be desirable that they be validated by autopsy studies. A more reliable distinction might be obtained by using electro-encephalography, computerised axial tomography, or nuclear magnetic resonance. Such techniques, however, would increase considerably the cost of a drug trial.

Assessment of Efficacy

Once patients fulfilling the diagnostic criteria for a study have been identified, consideration has to be given to defining criteria of therapeutic efficacy. As far as relatives and society in general are concerned, the most serious aspect of dementia is disturbed behaviour. Any assessment of efficacy should measure, therefore, behaviour which is (1) a source of worry or distress to the patient or his supporter; (2) is likely to be directly related to the pathology under study; (3) is unlikely to be the result of external influences; and (4) cannot be controlled by treatment currently available.

Other ways of measuring a response to treatment might include the measurement of biochemical changes in the cerebrospinal fluid or a brain biopsy, but there would be major ethical objections to this. Again, changes in electro-encephalographic patterns might be used, but the evidence is that this would not be sufficiently sensitive to pick up minor alterations in function. A wide range of tests used to measure cognitive function are available, but there is the objection that a statistically significant change in a test score may be of little practical significance in the management of a patient. Finally, the drug trial might well look at non-cognitive aspects of a dementia such as its effect on gait or the frequency of falls.

Selection of Subjects

Multiple pathology is so common in old people living in residential homes or long-stay wards that analysis of drug efficacy might be impossibly complicated. There would, therefore, be advantage in studying old people with dementia still living at home. A further advantage of this group is that many subjects would have relatively mild dementia, at which stage drugs might be expected to be more effective in preventing further deterioration. The problems involved in identifying such patients in general practice would be enormous, as would be the difficulties involved in ensuring compliance and in collecting accurate information on changes in behaviour from such a widely scattered population.

Duration of Assessment

An agent effective in the control of dementia may take a long time to work. A study therefore would have to extend over months or even years before a late response to treatment could be excluded.

Drugs Used in Dementia

While none of the drugs used to improve cognitive function have had a dramatic effect in elderly patients, it is important that these should be reviewed. This gives information on areas of research explored and found wanting, and on the other areas showing signs of promise where future work might produce major developments.

Vasodilators

The rationale behind their use in dementia is that patients with both Alzheimer's disease and multi-infarct dementia have a reduction in cerebral blood. An improvement in this might be expected to deliver increased quantities of oxygen to anoxic neurones.

There are theoretical objections to this argument. In Alzheimer's disease the diminished blood supply is the result rather than the cause of neuronal destruction, so that surviving neurones probably are adequately oxygenated. Many neurones in multi-infarct dementia are inadequately oxygenated, but these are adjacent to vessels blocked by atheroma and thrombus. Vasodilation occurs primarily in vessels unaffected by atheroma, so that blood would be shunted away from the ischaemic areas. Mental function, therefore, far from improving, might be expected to deteriorate. Drugs with a primary vasodilator effect tried in dementia include cyclandelate, papaverine, isoxuprine, cinnarizine, and betahistine.

Cyclandelate.   This is a vasodilator with three times the potency of papaverine. A large number of studies have been reported, some of which have suggested an improvement in cognitive function in both demented and alert elderly patients. It also increases cerebral blood flow, and produces electro-encephalographic changes. However, in a carefully designed study which included clinical ratings, a battery of psychometric tests, cortical evoked potentials, and the sedation threshold, results suggested that cyclandelate has no advantage over placebo in elderly patients with mild or moderate mental impairment.

Papaverine.   Papaverine is an extract of crude opium which relaxes smooth muscle arterioles. Most studies have suggested that it is of no value in Alzheimer's disease or multi-infarct dementia.

Isoxuprine.   This dilates cerebral blood vessels by stimulating beta-adrenoceptors. None of the properly controlled studies on it have produced evidence that it improves cognitive function in patients with mental impairment.

Cinnarizine.   This is an antihistamine with a vasodilator effect. It is of value in vertigo related to labyrinthine ischaemia, but there is no evidence that its effect on intracerebral vessels is of any value in mental impairment.

Betahistine. Though this drug is a histamine agonist it also produces cerebral vasodilation. In one study it produced an improvement in several tests of cognitive function and in functional capacity which was significantly greater than that for placebo. The authors suggested that a longer controlled trial should be performed to confirm or refute their findings. Experience with earlier cerebral vasodilators suggests that such a trial would be more likely to refute rather than confirm evidence of clinical improvement.

Vasodilators and Cerebral Stimulants

Some drugs, in addition to acting as vasodilators, also modify cerebral metabolism. It is suggested that by increasing the utilisation of oxygen by neurones they will improve cerebral function. Drugs with this effect include dihydroergotoxine, naftidrofuryl, and pentifylline.

Dihydroergotoxine. This ergot alkaloid derivative dilates cerebral blood vessels. It also has a complex effect on neuronal metabolism, in which it inhibits noradrenaline-stimulated adenyl cyclase activity and phosphodiesterase activity. Inhibition of adenyl cyclase responsible for cyclic adenosine monophosphate (AMP) formation prevents the cyclic AMP concentration from becoming excessive, while inhibition of the cyclic AMP metaboliser phosphodiesterase prevents cyclic AMP levels from falling too low. Dihydroergotoxine thus economises in cyclic AMP turnover, allowing the neurone to maintain a steady state in situations of stress such as anoxia.

Most studies have confirmed that dihydroergotoxine produces a statistically significant improvement in both psychological and behavioural performance. However, such an improvement in clinical terms usually is only marginal. It usually is insufficient to allow patients in hospital wards to go home, or to produce a reduction of pressures on relatives looking after them. It may be that in many of the studies the drug was used too late in the disease and that an investigation of its efficacy in early dementia might yield more positive results.

Naftidrofuryl. Naftidrofuryl is a vasodilator which also increases cerebral oxygen consumption, glucose utilisation and adenosine triphosphate production. This could have advantages in situations such as cerebral ischaemia where both oxygen and glucose are in limited supply. It has been used widely in elderly patients with mental impairment. In one hospital study, demented patients treated with the drug showed an improvement in performance significantly greater than that for placebo when scales completed by nurse, occupational therapist, and physician were used. There was a wide variation in response, however, so that while many patients improved on naftidrofuryl, others deteriorated. This may well be a reflection of variations in the underlying pathology treated with the drug.

A later study in general practice suggested that naftidrofuryl gave practical benefit to many of the patients treated. After treatment they often performed more household chores, looked after themselves better, coped better with shopping, and involved themselves in a greater range of recreational activities.

Surprisingly, patients showing this improvement showed no parallel improvement in tests of cognitive ability. Most studies, then, suggest that the drug may be of use in patients with mental impairment. A more difficult thing to quantify, however, is the extent to which this makes life easier for patients, relatives, and health professionals.

Pentifylline. This drug has a structure similar to caffeine and is bound to nicotinic acid. In addition to dilating blood vessels and having a stimulant effect it also increases cerebral glucose uptake. Further evaluation is required to establish the efficacy of this drug.

Cerebral Stimulants

There are several drugs which modify cerebral metabolism but do not dilate blood vessels. These include meclofenoxate and pyritinol.

Meclofenoxate. Evidence that meclofenoxate might be useful in dementia is the observation that it causes a decline in lipofuscin (age pigment) granules in neurones. At a biochemical level is increases glucose-6-phosphate dehydrogenase activity, thus promoting anaerobic metabolism. This is reflected in an enhanced resistance of cerebral cells to oxygen deprivation.

It improves mental performance in old people with mental impairment. This is related to an improved capacity for consolidating new information in the long-term memory store (Marcer and Hopkins 1977). Unfortunately, the practical benefits of this interesting effect have not been followed up by further trials.

Pyritinol. This drug also has a beneficial effect on nerve cell metabolism. It is reported as improving performance and behaviour in senile dementia. Further work is required to establish the clinical relevance of this. At present it is not in use in the United Kingdom.

Substrate Replacement

Acetylcholine. The dramatic response of patients with Parkinson's disease to dopamine deficiency has encouraged biochemists to investigate enzyme and substrate deficiencies in other neurological disorders. In Alzheimer's disease, abnormalities of acetylcholine metabolism have come under particular scrutiny.

Cholinergic neurones take up both acetylcoenzyme A and choline, which are combined by choline acetyltransferase to form acetylcholine (Fig. 11.1). This is released at the nerve terminal to be taken up by postsynaptic receptors, where it remains until it is metabolised by acetylcholinesterase to choline and acetate. In Alzheimer's disease there is a specific reduction in the amounts of choline acetyltransferase and acetyl-cholinesterase in cholinergic cells within the cerebral cortex. Though the changes are widespread they are most marked in more primitive parts of the cortex such as the hippocampus. The pattern differs

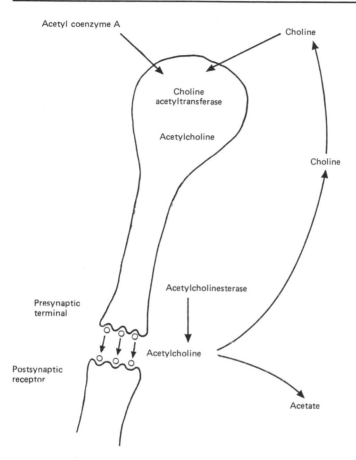

Fig. 11.1. Acetylcholine metabolism in the brain.

from that found in the brains of alert old people. Here there is a decline in choline acetyltransferase concentrations and a reduction in the number of acetylcholine binding sites, but no change in acetylcholinesterase activity. This could be interpreted as evidence that, in Alzheimer's disease, there is a selective dysfunction or loss or cortical cholinergic neurones. In "normal" ageing the biochemical pattern would fit that for a loss of all types of cortical neurones.

Evidence of specific acetylcholine deficiency in Alzheimer's disease has prompted investigators to try various forms of replacement therapy. Acetylcholine itself cannot be given because it is metabolised rapidly. An anticholinesterase might be effective by reducing acetylcholine breakdown in the cerebral cortex. Unfortunately, most anticholinesterases have severe peripheral nervous system side-effects, which include vomiting, colic, diarrhoea, and muscle twitching. What would be required would be an anticholinesterase with predominantly central effects.

Another option would be to give an acetylcholine precursor. Initial trials of choline in small numbers of severely demented patients have been disappointing. Large doses, say 9 g/day, may cause side-effects which include gastrointestinal discomfort, urinary incontinence, and depression.

The choline precursor lecithin (phosphatidyl-choline) is a more effective way of increasing blood choline levels, but there is no evidence as yet that it is any more effective than choline at improving mental function. Another precursor, deanol (2-dimethylamino-ethanol) also has been used in dementia, but again the results have not been encouraging.

Large trials incorporating guidelines mentioned earlier in this section are indicated. There is, however, the possibility that the enzyme deficiency in Alzheimer's disease is an epiphenomenon which is not related directly to impaired mental function.

Dopamine.   There is no evidence that patients with Alzheimer's disease have dopamine deficiency. It is surprising, therefore, that in a small double-blind crossover trial in patients with senile dementia, levodopa produced a statistically significant improvement in intellectual rating, communication, and continence (Lewis et al. 1978). If levodopa is used in Alzheimer's disease, it should be used with caution, since, far from improving cognitive function, it often induces an acute confusional state.

Tranquillisers, Sedatives, and Hypnotics

These drugs have already been described in detail. They have an important part to play in controlling some of the more distressing behavioural disturbances associated with dementia. It is important, however, that they are not used as a substitute for the careful assessment of a patient's problems. He may be distressed by the move to a strange environment, and here painstaking reassurance may be more effective than a large dose of haloperidol. Again, he may be agitated by a distended bladder. Here an enema or a bladder catheter is better than sedation.

If, despite assessment, a patient remains agitated, tranquillisers should be used, starting with thioridazine and going on to chlorpromazine if this does not work. More potent, but more disabling drugs should be reserved for situations where all else has failed. Benzodiazepines should not be used during the day as tranquillisers in demented patients. They often produce disinhibition rather than relaxation.

Hypnotics used for nocturnal wanderers should have a short duration of action so that they do not produce drowsiness the next day. Suitable hypnotics include chlormethiazole, the chloral derivatives, and short-acting benzodiazepines.

If, despite these, a patient remains agitated at night, it is worth using a single evening does of phenothiazine, say 50–75 mg thioridazine or 50–100 mg chlorpromazine. This may control nocturnal agitation and, at the same time, obviate the need for a tranquilliser the following day.

It should be recognised that demented patients may need to rise at night to pass urine. Over-enthusiastic nocturnal sedation may make a patient sleep through incontinence, or get up and fracture his hip. Sedation is no substitute for sensible, patient, and understanding nursing care on the part of relatives and professionals.

References

Isaacs B (1979) The evaluation of drugs in Alzheimer's disease. Age ageing 8: 1–7
Lewis C, Ballinger BR, Presley AS (1978) Trial of levodopa in senile dementia. Br Med J 1: 550
Lloyd-Evans S, Brocklehurst JC, Palmer MK (1978) Assessment of drug therapy in chronic brain failure. Gerontology 24: 304–320
Marcer D, Hopkins SM (1977) The differential effects of meclofenoxate on memory loss in the elderly. Age Ageing 6: 123–131

12 Terminal Care and Long-Term Care

In describing the management of terminal illness it is important that the condition should be defined (Table 12.1). People may die from a road traffic accident, from a cardiac arrest, or from a massive subarachnoid haemorrhage, and here resuscitative techniques receive priority. More often, they die during an acute exacerbation of a chronic condition, say, congestive cardiac failure or chronic bronchitis. Here again, attention is directed at saving life, and then stabilising the disorder. Other patients die at the end of a long crippling illness such as rheumatoid arthritis or a hemiparesis. Even with advanced disability, however, a patient may have a reasonable quality of life, so that simple palliation may be inadequate and measures designed to improve mobility or extend life often are indicated. Patients with advanced organic brain disease pose particular ethical problems, but even here, before he decides to withhold life-saving treatment, a clinician should be reasonably certain that, from the point of view of the patient, continued existence has no meaning or is intolerable. This leaves patients with a disease which is progressive, cannot be reversed by treatment, and which is almost certain to cause death within a period of days, weeks, or months. Many, but by no means all, forms of malignant disease fall into this category, as do neurological disorders such as motor neurone disease.

Table 12.1. Modes of death

1. Sudden death
2. Death during exacerbation of chronic disease
3. Death following a period of severe physical incapacity
4. Death following a period of severe mental incapacity
5. Death at the end of a progressive disease, e.g. malignancy or neurological disease

Once a terminal illness has been identified, the symptoms caused by it should be analysed in detail and treated appropriately. These often include pain, anorexia, nausea, vomiting, constipation, diarrhoea, thirst, dysphagia, breathlessness, incontinence, bleeding, and discomfort from pressure areas. Anxiety, confusion, depression, and insomnia often are concomitants of physical symptoms. An alternative is to say that nothing more can be done and give large doses of narcotics for all patients with a terminal illness. An even worse approach is to wait until the patient complains and then treat empirically the symptom described.

Pain

In terminal cancer the automatic response to pain may be to prescribe an analgesic, despite the fact that a wide range of conditions other than the tumour may be responsible for the pain. Examples include dyspepsia due to a hiatus hernia or peptic ulcer; discomfort due to a pressure sore; back pain due to osteoporosis or osteoarthritis; suprapubic discomfort from cystitis; or limb pain due to a poor peripheral circulation. Even if the tumour is responsible, active treatment may be indicated if this is likely to relieve symptoms. Examples are the use of corticosteroids in a headache due to a cerebral tumour; radiotherapy to a bony secondary; or cytotoxic therapy for a Pancoast's tumour.

Even when analgesics are considered to be the appropriate remedy for pain, it should be recognised that a wide range of factors influence the pain threshold of a patient. Someone who has slept badly, is tired, is frightened or worried, is lonely, or is depressed is more likely to be upset by pain. Past experience of a similar pain, or the outcome of a similar illness in a relative also influences the pain threshold. Conversely, a pain may not feel so bad if the patient has had a good night's sleep, has sympathy and support, understands what is going on, and has things to interest him and elevate his mood. The general management of the dying patient, then, often is as important as specific analgesics in the relief of pain.

There are several important general principles in the use of drugs for chronic pain. The first is that the dose of the analgesic be large enough to relieve the pain completely. Discomfort associated with an inadequate dose is likely to reduce the pain threshold further and ultimately result in the need for a much larger dose of analgesic. Again, the drug should be given regularly rather than on demand. A patient who has to ask for analgesics experiences frequent episodes of pain and, again, has a reduced pain threshold. In this context, it is equally important that the drug be given sufficiently frequently to avoid the recurrence of pain. Counting the minutes until the next dose or injection accentuates the severity of symptoms. Lastly, it usually is desirable that treatment which relieves pain should not cloud consciousness. The patient is then able to retain contact with his family, deal with his personal affairs, and indulge in recreation.

Morphine and Diamorphine

If a patient with terminal illness has severe chronic pain, morphine is the drug of first choice. Unless he is unable to swallow, this should be given orally, usually as an elixir (Table 12.2). The traditional Brompton cocktail also contains cocaine. This produces a temporary increase in alertness, but this is poorly sustained and is of little value in the long-term management of pain.

Table 12.2. Morphine elixir

Morphine hydrochloride	5 mg
Alcohol (90%)	0.625 ml
Syrup	1.25 ml
Chloroform water	5 ml

Note: Many hospital pharmacies produce morphine elixir with graded strengths of morphine so that it is possible to give much larger doses of morphine, e.g. 100 mg, in a small volume.

In terminal illness the starting oral dose of morphine should be 5 mg given every 4 h, waking the patient up at night if he experiences pain first thing in the morning. At 2-day intervals the four-hourly dose can be increased by 5-mg increments up to a maximum dose of 100 mg four-hourly. It may be that increasing morphine medication even at this rate is insufficient to keep pace with the pain. A solution to this is to give the patient a supply of 5-mg methadone tablets, instructing him to take one every time he experiences pain. As the dose of morphine increases the need for methadone declines, until at an adequate dose of morphine the patient is no longer taking methadone.

Patients may be troubled by having to take analgesics every 4 h, particularly overnight. This has led to the preparation of morphine in a slow-release matrix. If morphine is given orally in this form, plasma levels high enough to sustain analgesia are sustained for up to 12 h.

Given orally, diamorphine is absorbed more effectively than morphine, but the difference is of little practical importance. Diamorphine, however, is more soluble than morphine, so that larger quantities can be given by injection in the same volume of water. Injections should be reserved for patients who are unable to swallow or who have anorexia, nausea, or vomiting.

The administration of morphine and diamorphine carry with them real and theoretical penalties. Massive doses cause drowsiness and impairment of consciousness, but this effect wears off if the doses are continued. The problem can be minimised by starting with a small dose and gradually building it up. Again, patients may adapt to the drugs so that they no longer work as analgesics. This happens where dosage is increased only in response to intolerable pain. Tolerance does not develop if the initial dose is sufficient to prevent the patient experiencing pain, so that there is no need for him to request a larger dose.

Morphine and diamorphine often cause nausea and vomiting. In oral treatment the problem is resolved by adding 6.25 mg chlorpromazine to each 5 ml of morphine mixture. If injections are necessary a mixture of 50 mg cyclizine with 10 mg diamorphine may be useful.

Constipation is an inevitable concomitant of morphine or diamorphine therapy. In many situations the combination of a stool softener, say sodium sulphosuccinate 100 mg twice daily, and a stimulant laxative, say sodium picosulphate 10 mg daily, may be effective. The physiological advantages of bran as a laxative are balanced by the difficulty which terminally ill patients experience in taking it.

Narcotics are powerful depressants of the respiratory centre. Clinicians often are faced with the dilemma of treating intractable pain in a patient with bronchopneumonia or chronic obstructive airways disease. There is a considerable risk that if such a patient is given diamorphine or morphine he will die. Many doctors believe that in this situation their primary duty is to relieve pain rather than to preserve life at all costs. There is a clear ethical and legal distinction between this approach and using a massive dose of morphine in a terminally ill patient whose symptoms could be relieved by simpler and safer means.

The major problem of morphine and diamorphine, that they are drugs of addiction, has little relevance in a terminal illness.

Old people show an increased susceptibility to the effects of morphine and diamorphine. This should be borne in mind during the pre- and postoperative management. It is less relevant in terminal illness, where the dosage of analgesics is monitored closely against their efficacy and side-effects.

Alternatives to Morphine and Diamorphine

Both levorphanol and phenazocine have an analgesic potency which is three times greater than diamorphine. Levorphanol has no other particular advantages over morphine and diamorphine, but phenazocine has a longer duration of action, so that it can be given six-hourly rather than four-hourly.

Methadone is a drug which is equipotent to morphine but has a plasma half-life of 25 h. This means that repeated doses almost certainly would produce cumulation. There thus would be difficulty in using it in regular doses to relieve the pain of terminal cancer. The situation would be worse in old people where impaired hepatic metabolism would attenuate further its long half-life.

More recently developed alternatives to morphine and diamorphine are buprenorphine and butorphenol. Buprenorphine has about 25 times the potency of morphine, and about twice the duration of analgesic effect. The potency of butorphenol is about five times that of morphine, and it has a duration of analgesic effect of around 6 h. Neither drug has been evaluated in the management of chronic pain, but their longer duration of action suggests that they might have marginal advantages over morphine and diamorphine in this situation.

Where chronic pain is not severe enough to warrant morphine or diamorphine, papaveretum or dipipanone with cyclizine may be used. Though less potent than the former they possess all of their side-effects, including dependency, so that doctors should not be tempted to use them for chronic pain which is not associated with a terminal illness.

Pethidine and pentazocine also have been used as analgesics intermediate between paracetamol and morphine and diamorphine. Taken orally, pethidine has only a weak analgesic effect. Given parenterally, it has a duration of action of only 2–3 h. It also has little of the valuable euphoriant effect of morphine. Oral pentazocine again is only a week analgesic. It has the further disadvantage of inducing visual and auditory hallucinations. This makes it particularly unsuited to sick elderly patients, many of whom already have some degree of disorientation and confusion.

If pain is even less severe, even weaker morphine derivatives may be used. Dihydrocodeine has one-sixth the analgesic efficacy of morphine, and codeine one-twelfth. Dextropropoxyphene, a compound related to methadone, is usually formulated along with paracetamol (Distalgesic). Its analgesic efficacy lies between that of codeine and dihydrocodeine. A narrow therapeutic index means that it fairly frequently causes drowsiness, respiratory depression, and constipation. It also has a euphoriant effect which may be useful in terminal illness, but may cause dependency in patients with chronic pain of less sinister origin. Though popular with patients because of its euphoriant effects, it is probably overused in the elderly at present.

Patients with mild pain may respond to paracetamol alone. Large doses of aspirin are often surprisingly effective in the pain of terminal cancer. This may be related to suppression of prostaglandin synthesis enhanced initially by the malignancy. Doses of up to 1200 mg four-hourly have been recommended in young adults, but it is probable that this would produce intolerable side-effects in older patients. Nonetheless, a trial of salicylates, in enteric form, often can be justified before resorting to morphine or diamorphine.

Anxiety and Depression

Anxiety reduces the threshold for pain and may thus increase the need for analgesics. Patient and sympathetic counselling, as part of a well planned care programme, is the best way of alleviating anxiety, but there are times when this is not enough and drugs have to be used. Chlorpromazine probably is the agent of choice, and indeed is often given as an elixir in combination with morphine (see above). Sedation should be sufficient to allay anxiety, but not enough to depress consciousness to a level where the patient is unable to converse with friends and relatives or take part in day-to-day activities.

As in other situations, benzodiazepines are best avoided as tranquillisers in the elderly since they often accentuate agitation and confusion. Insomnia should be treated along the lines described in Chap. 11. It is worth reiterating, however, that by far the best hypnotic is effective relief of pain.

It might be thought that patients with a terminal illness do not survive long enough to develop a profound depressive illness and that the euphoriant effect of narcotics prevents this happening. Neither of these propositions is borne out by clinical experience. Many patients are depressed and live long enough to benefit from antidepressant therapy. Details of this are given in Chap. 11. Terminal illness, however, further compromises limited liver function in an elderly patient, so that it is wise to start on a low dose. Amitriptyline, for example, should be started at 50 mg daily.

Respiratory Symptoms

Coughing

A bronchial carcinoma may be accompanied by a persistent cough. A codeine or pholcodeine linctus is often effective. If the patient also has severe pain, the narcotic analgesic necessary to relieve this often also controls the cough.

Breathlessness

The management of breathlessness in the dying patient often presents considerable ethical and practical problems. If a patient is breathless as a result of obstruction of a major bronchus with a carcinoma, many doctors would be happy to control breathlessness with an appropriate dose of morphine. If, however, the breathlessness is due to a malignant effusion, drainage of the effusion followed by local cytotoxic therapy might be more appropriate. The situation might be rather different, however, if pleural secondaries were invading the thoracic cage and causing severe pain.

There again is the dilemma of how to manage bronchopneumonia developing during the course of a terminal illness. Whether this is treated with antibiotics depends on the condition of the patient. If it has developed late on in a long painful illness, if the patient is semi-comatose, and if the quality of life over the past few days has been deplorable, antibiotics should be withheld and his level of consciousness allowed to sink yet further. Conversely, if the patient may reasonably have been expected to live for a few more months, is relatively free of pain, has obviously been enjoying contact with his relatives, and is severely distressed by the dyspnoea, he should be given antibiotics. Unfortunately, the issues rarely are as clear-cut as in these two examples. Decisions on treatment should only follow careful discussion amongst medical and nursing staff, with relatives, and, where possible, with the patient.

A similar situation is breathlessness due to congestive cardiac failure. Here the relationship between the terminal illness and the cardiac failure is more likely to be coincidental, so that, more often than not, active therapy is indicated.

Urinary Incontinence

Confusion, immobility, faecal impaction, and urinary infection often result in a terminally ill patient becoming incontinent of urine. At this stage investigation by incontinence charts, urography, and cystometry and treatment with toilet training, anticholinergic drugs, and marsupial pants is likely merely to add to his misery. A more appropriate response is simply to control the incontinence by inserting a catheter. Long-term problems of chronic cystitis, pyelonephritis, and renal failure are irrelevant.

Alimentary Symptoms

Dysphagia may be due to neurological disorders such as motor neurone disease with bulbar palsy, or cerebrovascular disease with pseudobulbar palsy. The oesophagus itself may be obstructed by a carcinoma of oesophagus, stomach, or bronchus, or by enlarged hilar lymph nodes. In some instances palliative surgery is required to allow the patient to take nutrients, while in others it may be possible to pass a nasogastric tube. Few patients tolerate the standard nasogastric tube for more than a few days, but a fine-bore tube used in enteral feeding is much more acceptable. The content of the nutrients passed down the tube depends on the condition of the patient. In the terminal phases of his illness it usually is appropriate to correct dehydration, and pay less attention to protein, carbohydrate, and fat intake. If the patient is barely conscious, even fluid replacement may not be indicated.

Many patients with terminal illness suffer from anorexia, nausea, and vomiting. The treatment of this depends upon its cause (Table 12.3). Whenever possible, treatment of the underlying condition is preferable to complicating treatment with an anti-emetic. Examples are that faecal impaction can be treated with an enema, hypercalcaemia with corticosteroids, and drug-induced vomiting by stopping the offending agent.

If the condition is irreversible there is a wide range of anti-emetics to choose from (Table 12.4). Hyoscine is an effective anti-emetic, but its effect of reducing salivary flow limits its value in long-term treatment. It also reduces mucus secretion by the respiratory tract, and thus may be of use in a patient with a terminal respiratory rattle. Unfortunately, it often makes old people confused and restless, and thus is best avoided in them.

Though metoclopramide has an effect on midbrain chemoreceptor centres, its main action is to enhance peristaltic activity by stimulating postganglionic terminals in the gut wall. It is particularly useful where there is local gastrointestinal irritation. Though effective in radiation sickness it has surprisingly little effect on vomiting due to cytotoxic drugs. It causes drowsiness, but this is mild, so that it often is used in terminal illness where it is desirable that the patient be kept as alert as possible.

Chlorpromazine has a central anti-emetic effect and is particularly useful if the patient is anxious. If sedation is not desirable, trifluoperazine is an effective alternative. Prochlorperazine, perphenazine, and thiethylperazine also are anti-

Table 12.3. Causes of vomiting in terminal illness

Gastric irritation	Carcinoma, stress ulcer
Gastric obstruction	Carcinoma of pylorus
Intestinal obstruction	Carcinoma of bowel
	Faecal impaction
Metabolic disturbance	Uraemia
	Hypercalcaemia
	Carcinomatous toxins
Infections	Pyelonephritis
	Bronchopneumonia
	Pressure area
Drugs	Morphine and diamorphine
	Anti-inflammatory analgesics
	Antibiotics
	Iron supplements
	Potassium supplements
	Digoxin
	Levodopa

emetics, but are more likely to cause extrapyramidal symptoms than the first two preparations.

Cyclizine acts on the midbrain and, in terminal illness, is usually encountered when used in combination with an injection of morphine (Cyclomorph). There have been no studies comparing the relative efficacies of phenothiazines and

Table 12.4. Anti-emetic drugs

Agents	Oral dose
1. Anticholinergic agents	
Hyoscine hydrobromide	300–600 mg four times daily
2. Metoclopramide	10 mg three times daily
3. Phenothiazines	
Chlorpromazine	25–50 mg three times daily
Trifluoperazine	1–2 mg three times daily
Prochlorperazine	5–25 mg as required
Perphenazine	4 mg three times daily
Thiethylperazine	10 mg three times daily
4. Antihistamines	
Cyclizine	50 mg three times daily
Meclozine	150 mg as required
Dimenhydrinate	50–100 mg three times daily

antihistamines in terminal illness. At present, however, most clinicians use the former in preference to the latter.

Immobility, dehydration, weakness, and narcotic analgesics combine to produce severe constipation and faecal impaction in terminal illness. This often is a source of considerable distress, and requires careful investigation and treatment. Details are given in Chap. 6.

Pressure Sores

Pressure sores occur where continuous pressure prevents the flow of blood through an area of skin, eventually resulting in devitalisation and necrosis. Where a sore is due simply to prolonged pressure, the outlook is good. Often, however, other factors may be involved (Table 12.5). Thus, endothelial damage, thrombosis, or an impaired immunological response to infection increases the risk of the skin becoming devitalised, infected and ulcerated. If a large artery is blocked, skin death is inevitable. Also, epithelial cells may be damaged in a moribund patient as part of a more general process of tissue death. While pressure is the most important cause of pressure sores, then, many other factors may be involved, and it is important to bear this in mind when managing them. Relief of pressure and local treatment are not enough if a systemic disorder has suppressed wound healing and control of infection.

Table 12.5. Factors other than pressure potentiating cutaneous and subcutaneous damage

Endotoxins
Metabolic acidosis
Dehydration
Burns
Recent surgery
Bacteraemia
Systemic infection
Hypoxia
Stasis
Immunological depression

Systemic Treatment

Wound healing does not occur if a patient is subnourished. If the haemoglobin is less than 10 g/dl this usually should be corrected rapidly by blood transfusion.

Milder anaemias due to subnutrition can be treated by giving the appropriate haematinic.

Protein deficiency may manifest itself as hypo-albuminaemia, peripheral oedema, muscle wasting, and failure of wound healing. Few patients in this situation tolerate a high-protein diet and, if this is considered to be of sufficient importance, it may have to be given as an enteral feed via a narrow-bore naso-gastric tube. The protein imbalance often is due to increased tissue catabolism, so that it would seem logical to use an anabolic steroid. Examples include parenteral nandrolone or oral stanozolol. There is little evidence, however, that they actually work in this situation. An interesting recent development is the use of naftidrofuryl, a drug which stimulates cellular metabolism and which may be effective in correcting a negative nitrogen balance. Much further work requires to be done, but it may be that in the future this drug could prove useful in stimulating healing in patients with subnutrition.

Zinc plays an important role in protein formation and cell proliferation, so that deficiency might be expected to delay wound healing. This has been demonstrated in zinc-deficient rats, which showed a decrease in the formation of collagen and non-collagenous protein in skin wound granulation tissue. Oral zinc sulphate has been used in the treatment of varicose ulcers, but not all clinical trials have shown this to be of benefit. The mineral also was used in an uncontrolled trial for the treatment of pressure areas in elderly patients. Here it appeared to accelerate healing. Further investigation is required to establish (1) whether the treatment really works; and (2) whether it works in patients with both low and normal zinc status. If zinc sulphate is used, it should be given in an oral dose of 220 mg three times daily.

Ascorbic acid is essential for collagen synthesis and wound healing, so that disabled patients with deficiency of this are at grave risk of developing pressure areas. Ascorbic acid supplements also may have a dramatic effect on the rate at which pressure areas heal. Since wound healing increases the demand for ascorbic acid, it is likely that patients with both low and normal levels of the vitamin will benefit from this treatment. There is debate about the appropriate oral dose of ascorbic acid, but one of 500 mg daily is effective in most patients.

A variety of metabolic disorders may also delay wound healing. An example is that the ulcers of diabetic patients are less likely to heal if blood glucose levels are poorly controlled. Again, uraemia often causes skin ulceration. It may be difficult to impose a low protein diet on sick elderly patients. However, they often are able to take Hycal, a high-carbohydrate, low-fluid, and low-electrolyte drink. If given as 17 ml twice daily it often will reduce the blood urea concentration and accelerate pressure area healing.

Anoxic tissues will not heal, so that it is obvious that bronchopneumonia or acute exacerbations of chronic obstructive airways disease must be treated.

Tissue perfusion is essential to tissue vitality and this will be reduced if there is massive oedema or if there is a reduced cardiac output. The correction of cardiac failure thus plays an important part in the management of pressure areas.

Local Treatment

Table 12.6 lists some of the many preparations used in the local treatment of pressure areas. This diversity suggests that this area of medicine has not yet emerged fully from the era of folk medicine. Many experienced nursing sisters have their own favourite remedies, and, in the Middle Ages, it is likely that their predecessors obtained equally effective results with bats' wings, newts' eyes, or the powdered bones of mummies. Recently, careful clinical research, collaboration with histopathology and the use of new diagnostic skills such as thermography and radiometry, have shed a great deal of light on this previously dark area, so that treatment has become increasingly based on scientific principles.

Table 12.6. Topical agents used in the treatment of pressure sores

Antibiotics	Sulphathiazole, penicillin, chlortetracycline, gentamycin, neomycin
Elements and simple compounds	Bismuth, zinc, gold, hyperbaric oxygen, ionised oxygen, titanium
Hormones	Tethelin, stilboestrol
Foams	Fibrin, gelatin
Plasma	Plasma with Peru balsam
Brine	
Enzymes	Papain—urea—chlorophyllin, trypsin, collagenase
Sugar	
Tannic acid	
Miscellaneous	Tragacanth, pectin, urea, insulin, Peru balsam, formaldehyde, benzoin, silicone, antacids, kanya

Large pressure areas usually contain large quantities of dead tissues and are infected heavily. Much of the necrotic material can be removed by forceps and scissors. The remainder is loosened by washing with chlorhexidine. After this a soak of the antiseptic cetrimide should be applied and covered with an occlusive dressing. This usually is changed daily and removes most necrotic tissue in about 2 weeks.

During this period there is the risk that endotoxins will be released into the systemic circulation. If there is a lot of necrotic tissue the organisms responsible are likely to be anaerobic, so that the patient should be given cover with metronidazole in a dose of 400 mg three times daily. If other organisms such as *Proteus* or *Pseudomonas* are grown then other, often more toxic, systemic agents may have to be used. Topical antibiotics should be avoided since they rarely are effective, often cause local hypersensitivity reactions, or result in overgrowth by more resistant organisms.

Once necrotic tissue has been removed, attention should be directed to promoting re-epithelialisation of the pressue area under optimal conditions. This is done by applying a mild antiseptic to prevent infection and then covering this with an occlusive dressing. A suitable preparation is 0.5% cetrimide in a water-miscible base (Cetavlex). Another is 0.5% povidine iodine applied as a spray (Disadine).

Chlorinated lime and boric acid solution (Eusol) for many years was widely used in the management of pressure sores. Its main merits were that it promoted debridement, and was a powerful antiseptic. Unfortunately, it was so powerful that it destroyed early epithelialisation, and encouraged the formation of granulomatous tissue. When a pressure area healed, it therefore left an extensive area of scar tissue. Rapid bacterial destruction sometimes also led to release of high concentrations of toxins into the systemic circulation, resulting in disseminated intravascular coagulation and acute renal failure. Finally, there is a danger that the absorption of boric acid from large pressure areas may give rise to boric acid intoxication. Most cases of this have been reported in infants and young children. It may be, however, that in sick old people with pressure areas, multiple pathology and polypharmacy masked signs of toxicity.

A wide range of proteolytic enzymes have been used successfully as desloughing agents. These, however, are expensive and have no particular merit over the desloughing techniques already described. Again, Debrisan, a hydrophilic dextran polymer, is of proven efficacy in mopping up both exudate and bacteria from a pressure area. Its limitation is that the wound first has to be desloughed, and that it is of no value once the wound is dry. Well conducted controlled trials have shown that it has a place in the healing of pressure sores. Unfortunately it is expensive, so that evidence is required to show whether it has major advantages over the techniques already described for healing pressure areas.

Since the blood supply to pressure sores often is impaired, there are theoretical attractions to delivering oxygen to the wound. Various techniques, including the use of hyperbaric oxygen, have been employed. However, the delivery techniques are of such complexity that they arc unlikely to find acceptance by most nurses, doctors, or patients. Even then, there is as yet no clear evidence that the treatment works.

Since large numbers of patients suffer from pressure sores it is likely that in the future many more preparations will be marketed. In this field doctors will be well advised if they follow scientific principles and use only agents with which they are thoroughly familiar.

Subject Index